Acclai
Eros: A Journey (

"Both of us found the book to be a
sexual woman with its trials and tribulations, as well as its pleasures.
Anderlini-D'Onofrio's writing style is exquisite, its Italian flavors and
expressions included. Her story will help all people deal with their own
sexual orientations and lovestyles. Both of us agree that once we began
reading the book we were unable to put it down."

—The late Fritz Klein, MD, Former Editor, *Journal of Bisexuality,*
and Regina Reinhardt, PhD, Psychotherapist

"Serena's book is a brilliant combination of transcultural experience,
political and theoretical insights, commentary on academia, a mother's
preoccupations, all of which are interspersed with lots of juicy Eros. I
loved it!!"

—Suzann Robins, CHT, MA, Holistic Educator and Activist;
Faculty at Bloomfield and Caldwell Colleges, New Jersey

"Captivating, bold, titillating, saucy, yet earnestly nuanced, even at
times taxing in her intellectual reach, the Gaia of this absorbing cross-
cultural, cross-sexual tale is a twentieth-century Moll Flanders reborn as
horny intellectual. A scholar of gender and sex, a hands-on healer, and a
mother, the narrator discovers that she is never more wisely or more
transcendently herself than when she thinks in and with the flesh in all
its transient heat and sweetness. Her vividly told, politically engaged
tale of loves lost and found (often in surprising places) traces new moral
ground in redefining our identities as sexual creatures, as minds inhabit-
ing polymorphously erotic bodies, ever in quest of a sacred fullness of being."

—Flavia Alaya, PhD, Author, *Under the Rose: A Confession*

Eros
A Journey of Multiple Loves

HARRINGTON PARK PRESS®

Titles of related interest

When Husbands Come Out: Their Words, Their Stories edited by Fritz Klein and Thomas Schwartz

Bi-America: Myths, Truths, and Struggles of an Invisible Community by William E. Burlison

Life, Sex, and the Pursuit of Happiness by Fritz Klein

Eros: A Journey of Multiple Loves by Serena Anderlini-D'Onofrio

Eros

A Journey
of Multiple Loves

08-25-13

Serena Anderlini-D'Onofrio

For Karin
with love
and all good wishes

HPP

Harrington Park Press®
The Trade Division of The Haworth Press, Inc.
New York • London • Oxford

For more information on this book or to order, visit
http://www.haworthpress.com/store/product.asp?sku=5526

or call 1-800-HAWORTH (800-429-6784) in the United States and Canada
or (607) 722-5857 outside the United States and Canada

or contact orders@HaworthPress.com

Published by

Harrington Park Press®, the trade division of The Haworth Press, Inc., 10 Alice Street, Binghamton, NY 13904-1580.

PUBLISHER'S NOTES
The development, preparation, and publication of this work has been undertaken with great care. However, the Publisher, employees, editors, and agents of The Haworth Press are not responsible for any errors contained herein or for consequences that may ensue from use of materials or information contained in this work. The Haworth Press is committed to the dissemination of ideas and information according to the highest standards of intellectual freedom and the free exchange of ideas. Statements made and opinions expressed in this publication do not necessarily reflect the views of the Publisher, Directors, management, or staff of The Haworth Press, Inc., or an endorsement by them.

This is a work of fiction. Names, characters, places, and incidents either are the products of the author's imagination or are used fictitiously, and any resemblance to actual persons, living or dead, business establishments, events, or locales is entirely coincidental.

Cover design by Marylouise E. Doyle.

Library of Congress Cataloging-in-Publication Data

Anderlini-D'Onofrio, Serena, 1954-
Eros : a journey of multiple loves / Serena Anderlini-D'Onofrio.
    p. cm.
  ISBN-13: 978-1-56023-571-2 (alk. paper)
  ISBN-10: 1-56023-571-3 (alk. paper)
  ISBN-13: 978-1-56023-572-9 (pbk. : alk. paper)
  ISBN-10: 1-56023-572-1 (pbk. : alk. paper)
  1. Anderlini-D'Onofrio, Serena, 1954—-Fiction. 2. Bisexual women—Fiction. I. Title.
PS3601.N427E76 2006
813'.6—dc22
                                                                                    2005010765

May this story be a portal to all the other beautiful stories that intertwine with it, and may this book help us create the better worlds we need. Knowledge is love.

To my lovers, and their lovers, and their lovers' lovers, and so on across the globe, and to all children and parents.

ACKNOWLEDGMENTS

Without the people in my life who have made it so vibrant and interesting with their infinite contributions this book would not exist or would not be worthwhile. I am grateful for all the joys, sorrows, moods, moments, lessons, hopes, wisdoms, disappointments, and intensities we've shared.

A special debt of gratitude is owed to the early readers of this work, including Suzann Robins, Regina Reinhardt, Flavia Alaya, Maria Pallotta-Chiarolli, and the late Fritz Klein. I am also grateful to my daughter, Paola Coda, and my brother, Luca Anderlini, for their wise advice. A belated message of special thanks goes to my late mother and father who raised me to believe in the impossible and inspired me with their beauty and love. My gratitude also goes to the partners who have accompanied me for a stretch of the road; to the interlocutors who have shared their thoughts with me; to the mentors who believed in me and supported me in the most difficult moments; to the professors and students with whom I've shared a bit of the way; and to the communities who have hosted me and made me feel one of their own, including the bisexual community of San Diego, the holistic-health community of Encinitas, and the polyamorous community of Loving More. My gratitude also goes to the transnational community of AIDS dissenters, to the émigré community of UC Riverside, to my current academic community at UPR Mayagüez, and to all the other academic communities in which I have participated. I would also like to thank my neighborhood friends, interlocutors, and extended family in Rome and vicinities.

Finally, much gratitude goes to Bill Palmer and Josh Ribakove, and to my publisher and all of its collaborators, including Rebecca Browne, MaryLouise Doyle, Peg Marr, and others who have been patient enough to see this book through.

CONTENTS

Part Three: Epilogue

Part One:
Erotic Journey

I
Émigrés

The "New World" turned out to be full of all its promises. My move functioned as a proverbial "new start" which granted forgiveness for my youthful mistakes. I had never believed in the separation of body and mind, which reminded me of Marilyn Monroe's suicide for it seemed to be the result of the world's disbelief that the power of her beauty was a form of intelligence. To my wonderment, in the "New World" being sexy was considered compatible with being fit for academic work. Indeed, the very result of that supposed sexiness, my baby and responsibilities as a parent, only made me more credible for they were viewed as motivations for me to do more. In 1981, at twenty-seven, I was part of the first generation of Italian women who embarked alone on our journeys to the New World. It was a step in the direction of a long process of hybridization out of which the boundaries of my eros would be radically transformed. Giulio, my not-quite-ex-yet, was a major enabler of my adventure for he graciously offered to take care of our daughter Sara for the first nine months during which I was going to be away.

Strong with joy and trepidation, I embarked toward my New-World destination in the academic system that represented the kind of knowledge that was regarded as truly scientific in those modern days. It was like being catapulted in an entirely different, often incomprehensible world, a lifestyle about which I had to learn so much that I felt like a newborn. As I gradually became accustomed to the high-desert climate of Southern California, I also acclimated to on-campus living at UC Riverside, a highly research-oriented university situated at the extreme eastern periphery of the LA metropolitan area. I remember being entirely unprepared for driving on the freeway system. The regular traffic flow baffled my expectation that I would have to work my way around other drivers' erratic behavior. I also thought

I had turned into a monster, since when I walked on campus young men passed me by without glancing at me or making comments on my sex appeal. I didn't consider myself a star, but thought I was noticeable nonetheless. In Rome, I had been accustomed to exchanging gazes with passersby of the opposite sex, a street game as pervasive as Italian men's passion for soccer. Now I missed that sense of living body-against-body, and being left alone felt like an abandonment rather than a liberation. Then I realized that there were places where men gazed, the downtown areas where cruisers paraded in their shiny cars, and the "meat-markets," bars where one went to get laid. Neither one of these matched my style, since my car was not something to show off, and I found the bars depressing.

Part of me was searching for a new mode of sexual play, so the fact that the Italian-American community was out of reach felt like a blessing. Fortunately, I spoke French, which gave me access to the émigré community that used that language. And that's where I met Stephane, finally the lover who was my peer, and someone my father, Dario, would approve of. He was the person with whom my heterosexual development culminated. With him I was going to have the relationship that turned out to be most difficult to process into a friendship in the light of later developments, precisely because it was based on equality and freedom both in intellectual and erotic expression, and in parenting.

As a teacher and student of many years, I know that, no matter what sexual-harassment policies say, learning is erotic since it activates the pleasure of discovery by putting brain cells in motion, and stimulates the body-mind by opening up new vistas and possibilities to the imagination. The erotic energy emanating from this process is what keeps people in schools—it is what keeps us engaged in the learning process, be it as students or as teachers. That this energy needs to be channeled in socially productive and acceptable ways is just as necessary as denying its existence is perverse. I was not fully aware of this when I first entered the classroom where I was going to teach my first course. But soon I was going to find myself in the perfect situation where falling in love with a student was not only permissible, it was even encouraged, and where I was going to become my student's teacher of language as well as of love. The eerie sense of omnipotence that this gave me had a price that was to be exacted later on.

Stephane was a shy student in broken Mexican sandals and knee-length corduroy shorts. He had silver-rimmed eyeglasses and slightly uncouth hair, with a rebellious lock overshadowing his eyebrows. His English had a thick French accent, and he was visibly out of place in the high-desert campus where we met, yet he was brave enough to stick through it and make things work. He was a graduate student and research assistant in soil and environmental sciences, and was taking Italian for his own contentment. We were about the same age, our mid- to late twenties, and I was just as incongruous in my white cotton shirt, wide-pleated skirt, and pumps. I did my act fairly well in the beautiful seminar room to which our Italian class had been assigned, with an enrollment of about twelve. When I asked around where students came from, none of the mentioned LA suburbs rang a bell. I didn't have the foggiest idea of what Pasadena, Monterey Park, Pomona, and Claremont were like, or how to get there. But I had heard of Stephane's birthplace, Paris, France.

He seemed a bit lonely and I thought I'd like to get to know him better. I asked some Algerian friends to organize a party and invited him. We danced, and he seemed a bit naïve for his age, a rookie, or somebody who could use a teacher in many ways. We left and rode our bikes home. A vernacular saying from the city of Rome, *fatta e magnata,*—make it and eat it—is used for things that are too good to be left for another day. Images of great foods like pasta al dente and hot cakes popped up in my head. How juicy and delicious when they are cooked and gulped down right away, but later, how quickly they become mushy and stale! We came to the crossroads where my way home and his diverged. We knew that I had a roommate and he didn't, as I hinted that we make the turn his way. He rented a nice room on university premises, in a wooden building with nifty landings and lofts. I found his decorations indulgent: the stained-glass lamp flooded the alcove with an aura of deep purple, a decadent flavor of French aristocracy mixed with bohemian artistic flare as we lay on the carpeted floor. I remember watching his naked body covered with hair, the pleasure of smelling and touching it in every detail. He was on the meaty side, with narrow shoulders, large hips, prominent chest almost feminine in shape, with an inspired, thoughtful face. The androgyny of his hairy breasts almost drove me crazy. I noticed how he relished my gaze. He was a blank slate, and I could finally pass my erotic lessons on to someone else.

We spent many hours in our love embrace, and then I exclaimed, "Now you have to drop my course, for I can't sleep with my students. Didn't you know?"

"No, I won't," he said. "I've decided to learn Italian and yours is the only course."

I was taken aback and made him swear he would pretend this episode never took place. The image of Gabrielle Russier, the French female teacher in Paris who had fallen in love with a student during the revolution of May 1968, and then committed suicide, kept popping up in my head. We heard about her in Rome, while we were having our own "May '68." The scandal was that the student was not a girl, the professor not a man. But they were in love, and her death became an emblem of how our revolution was right and necessary. *One sacrificial heroine is enough, though,* I reflected in my UC Riverside dorm. To assuage my anxiety, I decided to consult with the only female professor my department was fortunate to have.

"Going out with a fellow graduate student is perfectly okay," she reassured me to my astonishment, "even though he just happens to be taking your course. In fact," she suggested, "this relationship could be a good investment for all involved. If you two like being together, you'll be more successful and happier to stay in our programs."

I could not believe I deserved such happiness and congratulated myself on truly discovering a "new world."

"In case we continued our relationship," I said the next time I saw Stephane, "there will be no cheating whatsoever in the course, and no letting on that we are together while on campus, okay?"

I lived in the dorms, and after one semester a loft next to Stephane's place became available. I don't know how the system conspired to pander to our relationship, but, without asking, I moved in.

The shell of my "troubled child" identity was breaking to give birth to a new person. *What a great deal,* I thought. *In Italy I'm in a no-win situation where I'm either sexy and stupid, or ugly and nerdy. Sexy students are expected to sleep with professors, for lusty professors are always ugly and male. Sexy students are always pretty and female, and sexual harassment is not even a concept yet. If I am sexy and make good grades, then the burden of proof that I'm really earning them is on me, for, as the thinking goes, "It would be so much easier for her to get A's the other way."* In my experience, the Italian system made it impossible to upgrade girls like me from student to professor. Graduate degrees did not exist yet and teaching assistantships were unknown. The few young graduates who were asked to assist professors—in view of possible career developments—did it all without pay. Nor was there a way to find an instructor with whom sex could be fun, for, at least in the humanities, academics had to keep a reputation for being intellectuals, and a droopy body in shabby clothes was necessary. Now I get to be the teacher, and I'm obviously sexy. My favorite student only asks to make love to me, and this is considered great! Had I been able to design a New World for myself, I couldn't have asked for more. Obviously, the version of academic culture that prevailed in Southern California dealt me a generous hand. In the wider halo of Hollywood, a person's body and mind had to be handsome. Of course, I could not imagine what this culture would do to one who looked weak, sick, or old.

In the decadent dorm room, I'm a confidante to my new lover. "I've never really been with a woman before," Stephane admits one night as we lie in bed under the boudoir lamp.

"As an adolescent I was molested by an older man—a friend of my parents. He claimed to be a mentor who'd show me the wonders of geology. I was a very diligent boy." He proceeds to describe the enchanted world of his parents, full of lofts, studios, canvasses, colors, sculptures, paintings, and all the things that I, from a more conventional family, had always dreamed of. "My mom and dad are artists," he explains as he elaborates on the cozy intimacy of their bohemian lifestyle.

"The magic must have been bedazzling," I comment, as the thought of oil-paint odors and textures turns me on.

Stephane is accustomed to his parents' frugality and artistic devotion. "And yet," he explains, "I long for something more scientific—more sòlid. I've always done my homework, never cut class, never talked. I was almost too obedient, and my parents were worried that I would not truly have a rebellious, adolescent phase—that I would not go through the crisis that makes one a man. They told their friend, who proposed to help. 'I'll show the boy something he can enjoy,' he promised. The older man came to pick me up at the small apartment in the historical center," Stephane continues. "We went hiking in geologically interesting areas, and that's where he masturbated me to orgasm. We were in the fields, and I did not find it all that strange. At home, I was used to nudity from my parents' paintings. But of course I would not keep such a secret from them, and so the trips came to an end. I quit geology and never matured sexually."

I look at him puzzled. "Last time you did fairly well," I comment.

"Before you, my only experience with a girl was when my best friend's girlfriend agreed to have him watch us while I made out with her."

I think that being with a *fils d'art,* a child of artists, is wonderful, and don't mind a bit passing my lessons along. "I'll teach you everything I know," I reassure him.

Now our first Halloween party is going on. My new French lover knows that back in Italy, my quasi-ex husband, Giulio, is a Mardi-Gras cross-dresser. Stephane and I reinterpret American Halloween in a similarly transgendered way, with me showing up for the party in male drag, impersonating—with a bit of chutzpa—Rodolfo Valentino. I like the way I look in male attire. I feel excited and horny. My friends don't recognize me, and actually guess correctly as to whom I am disguised as. I feel I'd make a pretty appetizing male and enjoy the freedom of movement I have. Stephane is dressed as a doll, with ponytails and a pink dress clashing with his carved, angular face. He wears red lipstick and blush, his shoulder straps show a white, chubby chest covered with dark, curly hair. He is melancholic and campy. I can't help thinking that my quasi-ex Giulio, with his flat face and hairless body, makes more of a good-looking girl. But then this tells me that probably Stephane is the man my father, Dario, will approve of.

When dressed appropriately, we look like the perfectly gender-adjusted couple. We make a good-looking pair, I reflect. He is a bit taller than I am and with a slightly larger bone structure.

His masculinity is denoted by his arched nose and hairy chest, my femininity by my slender chin and long legs. The way we look as a couple reminds me of my parents. I get the feeling that keeping my centeredness while in this relationship will prove as difficult as giving up the relationship altogether.

Piqued with queer curiosity, Stephane and I visit San Francisco, the famed Mecca of gay culture, the city that, at least before the AIDS scare, held the promise to reveal everything to those curious about sex beyond the straight borders. We visit Castro with its displays of hyper-masculine gay men. "Not a bit of effeminacy," he observes. Not much lesbian culture on display, I notice. As provincial tourists from a small satellite town near LA, we reflect, "Wouldn't it be great to be part of this scene? So much to learn!" But both of us are foreigners with no working permits. Our student visas have been obtained based on the statement that all the activities in which we engaged before we came were neither homosexual nor communist in nature. "Are we now free to do what would warrant INS the right to send us back home?" We realize we are prisoners of the ivory towers that brought us here in the first place.

Back in Riverside, the sexual behavior the émigré community accepts is monogamous and monosexual. Sex happens between a male and a female and does not involve other sexual players. Good sex implies an exchange of pleasure that is both reciprocal and simultaneous. The "other" is both a person of the other gender, and the cosmos to which one becomes connected via erotic energy. On the sidelines, some self-pleasuring might be going on, but it is never discussed or acknowledged in a positive way. There is no understanding of the mere giving and taking of pleasure as erotic experiences in and of themselves, nor is there any awareness of how toys and other technologies might enter the game.

My bisexual impulses are sublimated in my interest for female writers. I can safely pursue it as a professional goal, for it is not emotional or sexual and so it does not threaten my straight identity. In the UC system, all existing books are held in the library and I can check them out any time I want. There are no apparent restrictions on pursuable objects of knowledge, hence, as I discover, one can study female characters and female writers as well.

I make a secret deal with the academic world: *I stay in this bankrupt system of male knowledge as long as I can subvert it at least enough to focus on women all my research energies,* I promise myself.

As a teaching assistant, I accept to teach male knowledge. In Italian, my students learn, all nouns have a gender. It's as if words were more sexy in a way. But the trick is, the default gender is male, so, for example, if in a group of girls there is just one boy, the whole group is masculine for grammatical purposes.

"Isn't this unfair?" Stephane asks from his nearby desk.

"Of course, but I'm not making the rules, just passing them on."

I split the teacher's persona from the researcher. The teacher belongs to the system, but as a graduate student, one better not ask me to have men be the subject of my research or I quit right away. The library frees me for I can point to respectable female writers whose books are there and about whom my male professors don't even know. They want to keep me in their graduate program, for they need me to teach their basic courses, so they let me do what I want. The horizon of my imagination expands. There is a year when I decide I'll only read books by women, just to get a sense of how it feels to be immersed in a female world. I bask in this new discursive space, even though, at some level I am still hooked on male energy—I believe that only males have the power of enabling me to become who I want to be.

As I started my life as an émigré, I found myself in an international community that was closely knit but culturally suspended between the Old and the New World. We lived on the American continent but had a European imaginary, which was confirmed and even made stronger by our presence to each other. We were everything to each other, for our families, and all the other people, things, and places that had been familiar since childhood were far away—even as they were ever present to our imagination. As a Francophone community, we shared an existentialist attitude toward the New World, which at times verged on hyper-realism, as in a book by Jean Baudrillard. It was a mixture of fascination and contempt, which really did not resolve the issue of why we were there in the first place. Our existentialism was a rejection of zeal and perfectionism, it was a response to the totalitarianisms that had swept our parents' worlds. Its emphasis was the individual and a human dimension, but as existentialists we overlooked integration within a larger whole, and our dependence on it for our life's work. Perhaps because we flaunted our lack of faith, be it in the system or in some divine force, a distance between the émigré community and white America was maintained. It was a mixture of mutual fear and lack of respect. It felt as if whites expected from us an ecstatic attitude toward the New World we were unwilling to deliver. Little did we know that they were past that attitude themselves, but were aptly trained in faking it and in counting on foreigners to do their dirty work. Things were different with African Americans, whom we admired for their role in the civil rights movement, and whose heroes we worshipped, including Angela Davis, Malcolm X, Martin Luther King, and Cassius Clay. African Americans were eager to get near us and valued our friendship, perhaps as a result of their memory for the respect encountered by black musicians and writers in Paris, even before their white compatriots bothered to notice their works. It was a way to bond with a kind of America that was not quite so fully persuaded of its own decency and right to exercise mastery over the rest of the world.

The part of the New World where we were stationed also offered access to a different dimension in the concept of nature. In the west, entire landscapes were still untouched by human endeavor. Visiting the wilderness and hiking the national parks put us in touch with a dimension of nature foreign to our European imaginary, every inch of the old continent being marked by a millennial human presence. In the nearby deserts one could access a sense of the earth as an embodied maternal being who was naked. Our scientifically oriented campus hosted a pioneer soil and environmental science department and scored high in environmental awareness. We knew how dangerous environmental pollution was, especially since Riverside received all the smog produced by LA, but we still saw the environment in relation to ourselves. A more holistic sense of ecology had not yet entered our consciousness and we did not see animals, plants, and minerals as beings with meanings and a purpose of their own. Our sexual practices, enhanced by the arts, and based on codependence of males and females, further marked our separation from a holier sense of embodiment and cosmic connectedness.

As a woman who had already had a baby, I was fortunate to enjoy the benefits of mechanical birth-control technology, for I could easily wear an intra-uterine device, or IUD. Since my uterus had already been inhabited by a long-term host, it was capable of tolerating a small metal spiral within itself. Its effect was that of saturating the intrauterine environment with copper, which rendered it inhospitable to newly fertilized eggs. For those able to wear them, IUDs were less risky than birth control pills, for they functioned mechanically and were not based on long-term use of hormones suspected of being carcinogenic. However, IUDs were not devoid of effects on the body's ecology. The lining of the uterus was often irritated, and this resulted in ongoing infections such as candidiasis. Their long-term effect was a reduction of the friendly bacterial flora that facilitate the absorption of nutrients by the body, a reduction that weakens the immune system. In my mechanistic knowledge of my own body, I was not aware of these problems, and welcomed the privilege of being at all times ready and available for unprotected sex. The free and complete exchange of fluids we enjoyed enabled Stephane and I to often experience previously unattained peaks of erotic ecstasy.

After the Halloween follies, we spent the year studying together, our social life revolving around Geraldine and José, a female and a male friend from Switzerland who were also together. I told Geraldine about Sara, my four-year-old daughter back in Italy waiting to join me. "I don't know how to break the news to my new boyfriend," I said one evening as we walked in the quad.

"Stephane loves children," she commented. "He volunteered at a child care center in Paris the year before he came."

"Then I can tell him?"

"He'd probably be excited to stepparent," she said softly as she smiled and cocked her head.

Geraldine turned out to be correct, and I found myself in a perfectly balanced emotional triangle, with a female friend and confidante on one side, and a male lover on the other. This arrangement reminded me of my high school days, when my friend Emanuela was my soul mate, and both of us engaged in sexual and erotic experiments with our respective boyfriends. José and Stephane were scientists, a biologist and a chemist respectively. Geraldine was a historian, and I was a literary person. It was such a perfectly balanced combination of intellectual and emotional energies that almost all areas of our creative intelligence could be fed. Our physiques were also similar. Both Geraldine and José looked European, with their elongated bodies, thin muscles, and long, wavy hair. Geraldine had more of a French flare, with brown eyes and a sculpted, delicate face. José was more of a German type, with blue eyes and blond hair. Stephane was dark and handsome like a romantic hero from France, and I was the sensual Italian with a long body and wavy hair. Not that there was no jealousy or competitiveness among us. For one thing, I was sometimes jealous of the confidence Geraldine and Stephane had. And, since I found José especially mature and handsome, I was a little envious of Geraldine for getting the best-looking guy. But overall these feelings were secondary and our friendship was so encompassing of our whole beings that we could have swapped partners any time, for our auras were melted anyway.

Throughout the first year of my stay, my student/lover learned Italian religiously, as the language that would soon give him access to our planned shared parenting. Major steps were taken also in our erotic development. I explored the woman-on-top position fully, and discovered the pleasure of having the head of a penis stroke over my labia and clitoral area. He learned to control his erection so that he would prolong his pleasure and I would always come first. I even got early hints of what was hiding in one of my closets, when we made love in our friends' bedroom, and I discovered that Geraldine's nude photographs turned me on.

When my daughter Sara joined us, in the second year of my stay, Stephane and I moved out of the single-student apartment complex and got a small family-student house of our own. Sara was a thin and feisty five-year-old, with wide green eyes and ubiquitous hands. We formed a great blended family, with three languages in use: Italian among us and the little girl, French between the two of us, and English among the three of us and the outside world. Our sleeping arrangements rotated between the two available bedrooms, so that each one of us would have a time with a whole bedroom to himself or herself. We were perfectly comfortable with our bodies and nudity in the home. Sexual activity was a little bit on the low end, since so much more was going on, but household and parenting chores were always shared.

It was at that time that the Riverside pollution became a serious concern. Close to the upper end of the major hydrological basin of Southern California, Riverside was about sixty miles east of LA, the metropolitan area that produced the carbon monoxide that sea winds blew toward us. Riverside's high-desert climate was favorable to orange groves and, in the early Hollywood days, the city had been a resort for stars in search of repose, with its dry, perfumed air. But as the metropolitan area grew—and as the train system was bought away by car companies—the exhaust gasses of the 4 million cars in circulation in the basin formed a huge cloud of a dusty brown color, and one could see its ominous volume take over the valley at around 10 a.m. As the smog set in, the buildings across the road looked wrapped in a thick light gray, brownish veil. In the winter there were a few clear days, when the north winds blew the smog away. The city had gradually been co-opted by the larger metropolitan area, and was now a commuter town and affordable residential area. Riversidians, of course, were innocent of any harm. All of us residents were victims of mal-development, proof of the kind of environmental degradation that can be produced by urban sprawl—especially when accompanied by inadequate public transportation. Rome, my birth city, is also in a bowl, but compactness and public transportation keep fuel use down. I had never questioned the faith my father, Dario, had in technological progress and the belief in modernity that still held sway in his world. But the ecological disaster of Southern California was way beyond my direst imagination. Being the powerless parent of a fragile creature entrusted to my care began to change my consciousness. Stephane and I did what was possible, and, as soon as school let out, we'd ship Sara back to Italy, in Bosa, the beach town where she stayed with her Sardinian relatives until her return in the fall.

The compound where we lived had belonged to the military. It was a park with willows and oaks; the campus a ten-minute walk away. The barracks had been turned into duplexes with diminutive rooms and low ceilings. The child care center was right next to our little home and one could see it from the kitchen window while sharing meals during which our cultural differences emerged. Stephane's idea of pasta was a mushy thing out of tin cans that parents serve before going out to dinner on their own. He had never learned to roll spaghettis, and I would not allow cutting them. Sara intervened, and taught him how to set a few apart on the edge of the plate, and wrap them around his fork, until the roll could be brought to his mouth without splurging. We often laughed about this amusing role reversal. Stephane was open to the hybridization and Sara felt proud of her bedrock Italian manners. Stephane always felt that both Sara and I had a strong ethnic community in which to belong, and of which he felt deprived as an expatriate from a major colonial power of the modern age.

When Sara came to California, Geraldine and José went back to Switzerland, and I became aware of erotic triangulations in romance and parenting. When Sara, Stephane, and I moved in together, I realized that for Stephane Sara was the gravitational force that made him stay. She was a third pole in the energy field between Stephane and myself, and it felt great that biology didn't matter. But I also felt this was unfair to Sara's dad. Sara was forgetting Giulio, and I was afraid this would alienate him further. I wanted to keep both parental options open for my daughter.

Geraldine and José returned to Europe in the fall of 1982. Before I arrived, the two of them and Stephane had been inseparable, Stephane functioning as Geraldine's confidante. They were so intimate one could have bet they were a triad. I completed the quadrangle, and everybody felt safe and happy, everybody's emotional and sexual needs being met in an acceptable way to the heterosexual world. Later, with Geraldine and José gone, I felt bereft and started having problems, both sexual and emotional, in my relationship with Stephane. He could not meet my emotional needs, and so even the sex became bad. I missed my female friend. I needed a triangle, and the third corner was gone. Back in Geneva, Geraldine was also very unhappy, had problems readjusting to Europe, and missed José who'd gone to Germany. And perhaps she missed Stephane and me as well—the intimacy the four of us had shared. I remembered Geraldine's bedroom and her nude photos plastered to the walls, when for the first time it had been in my face that a woman's body could turn me on.

That winter, Geraldine wrote us a letter about José. Her now long-distance boyfriend was going out with another woman. "He writes that both he and his girlfriend think they're gay, but too afraid to come out, and so they feel somehow imprisoned by this secret together," Stephane said as he read aloud from her letter. "I don't believe a word," Geraldine's letter continued. "This is just bullshit José made up to make me feel bad."

"I'm sure she's right," Stephane commented as he sat on the edge of the bed.

I took the letter in my hands and asked, "How can you be so sure? Maybe it's not bullshit. The guy could be just trying to be honest." I could see how, now that he had confessed his queerness to his new girlfriend, and she to him, their secret kept them together, at least until one decided to act on it.

Stephane looked upset. "I think José's wrong," he insisted, unable to even contemplate his own longing for that friendship.

Yet this biphobia would not keep us from playing gender-bending games. Campus culture was increasingly aware of rape, and Stephane and I could not help but notice that the rapist was always male, the raped, female. Both of us were proud of our egalitarian mentality and felt that this underestimated females. "There must be a way in which a woman can rape a man," I commented. And that's how we came to see our private erotic performances, especially those in which I was the initiator, as examples of male rape.

In the past, a respectable woman was supposed to say no, for she had been trained to do so to protect her reputation and her value as a marriage commodity. A woman's "no" meant that she was perform-ing well as a coy, feminine person—that she was playing hard to get. Alluring young men always presumed that their ability to arouse her senses would prevail on her intellect, and that, in the middle of their passionate love embrace her "no" would become so feeble as to turn into a "yes." Since most women did not receive any sexual education, and were unaware of how else their body could be pleasured, many times this was exactly the case. But now, in an attempt to fully and definitively regulate this highly subjective matter, sexual-harassment codes legally established that, no matter how, with whom, and where, "when a woman says no it means no." Would this mean that when a man says no it also means no? Indeed, when a woman's voice says no, it is hard to prove whether her body gives another message, for one cannot see what's happening inside her vaginal walls until one is in there. But when a man's voice says no, his body might be saying yes with a flamboyant erection. In this case, the man's genitals and his voice make two opposite statements. "Which one is more correct?" we wondered. In the past, rape had been a crime against the woman's family, often repaired with the rapist marrying the girl. Now rape was a crime against the person, and rightfully so, but then, the will and in-tent of the persons involved would have to be determined, rather than its mere verbal expression. Would this always be possible? I raped Stephane when his body responded to my pleasure to find his own pleasure in the surrender of his will to my desire. He raped me when he insisted on anal penetration and allowed it to happen slowly enough for my sphincter to open. But it is a "rape" for which I am grateful, for it made me discover one of the strongest orgasms I can have. These were totally consensual rapes, games symbolic of the erotic power we had over each other.

II

Triangulations

The presence of my baby girl in the émigré community of those early years in California kept my inner landscape free of existential anxiety. Sara was a cozy bundle of joy, and, as in the Italian motherly tradition of raising children, we had a very corporeal relationship, made of cuddling, hugs, rubs, kisses, and other body-to-body attachments, including occasional spanking. It was a two-in-one mode of being, based on the shared memory of her prenatal fusion with me. As I experienced the world through her body, we formed a holistic unit that participated in the existence of the earth as an animated being, something I was to later compare to the figure of two-in-one delineated by Irigaray in her famous essay, "When Our Lips Speak Together." The compound where we lived was reserved to family students, either single parents or regularly married. Sara received no child support from Giulio, but both Stephane and I saved by living together, and we had a comfortable, homey life as well.

There were four little girls just on our street, and they ran around outdoors all day. There were multiple ethnicities, nationalities, and races. Sharma was an African American from Chicago and LA, Monica a Latina from Argentina, and Kathy was the only white girl. We traded babysitting, and the children learned about cultural preferences. Macaroni and cheese was a staple, and Sara loved it, to my horror. Sara returned to Italy at age eight, and having grown up there, she has become an excellent cook of pasta entrees. "I am not American," she says when I speak English to her today. But when she visits me in North America, she drives me to the drugstore for a box of those mushy elbows wrapped in yellow cheese. Then she comes home and pigs out on them to her heart's content. "The taste of your childhood," I tease her, and remind her of the outdoor games and sense of freedom in space she developed in her Riverside years. There was a

magic correspondence between us and the universal harmony and order that created itself around us wherever we'd be.

Sara and I were positioned at the edge of a university system which
treated women's knowledge as ignorance. Knowledge was modeled
on war, an invasion of the field or body to be searched and conquered
by the knowing mind. But our presence brought in our sense of economy as subsistence, of ecology as balance in the energy fields between
related beings. We were a site of resistance to the mechanistic con-
cepts of learning, justice, and well-being generated by the prevalent
masculine epistemology. I remember Sara being always healthy,
happy, and full of energy. She had very few toys but was always busy.
Later on, when she became more insatiable and less appreciative, I
kept thinking back of this blessed time when ecological frugality was
the measure of a child's freedom and happiness. As the only child being raised within the Francophone émigré community, Sara was the
gravitational center for the kind of extended family that this community constituted. Based on our commitment to shared parenting,
Stephane and I created a home around her, and this space provided
stability and structure to others as well. Single women, or male-
female couples whose various origins fell within the areas affected by
the French colonial legacy, would refer to us for social life, conversation, excursions, or simply dropping in to say hello and share a meal.
They turned the two-in-one being formed by Sara and myself into a
center of gravity of its own.

During the 1983-1984 holidays I went to Europe on a research trip
and left Sara with Stephane. Eve was an environmental scientist from
France on a two-year fellowship new on campus that semester. She
was a Northern-European type, with straight blonde hair down to her
shoulders, an androgynous body, and long legs. I hoped she'd become
my friend, replacing Geraldine, and my high school mate Emanuela
before her, in her role of confidante and next best thing to a sister. Eve
had a deep, gravelly voice and there was something vulnerable and
earnest about her. But she was single, and I feared she would look
down on me as a woman devoted to parenting rather than professional success. The either/or logic that opposed career and parenting
loomed large, despite my efforts to be a model for a both/and alterna-

tive. Unattached women looked down on female parents, resenting the stigma attached to their own, less conventional choice. Having been on this side of the divide since my early twenties, I could not imagine that sense of superiority to be the other face of a lurking resentment.

Eve had already blended into the community but she gravitated around our house more than the others, which I interpreted as a need for a sense of family. I also found Eve sexually attractive—imagined how Stephane could be attracted to her. I felt the vibrations in the energy field between them, and wanted to be in it, yet didn't know how to interpret this response.

While I was away, Eve took on part of his duties as a substitute parent. Alone with each other, Eve and Stephane had a brief, intense fling they only ambivalently enjoyed, with me on their minds. When I returned I knew something was going on. Once more, Sara had catalyzed the energy and things happened around her.

But Stephane believed my love lesson that it was best to be discreet about one's affairs. We saw a counselor together, and after much prompting he confessed.

"It was hard while you were away," Stephane claimed, "and Eve helped."

"I knew she liked you," I replied. "I could feel it before you became aware of it." I wondered why Eve hadn't wanted to become my confidante. *Why has she chosen him over me? What did she feel about me?* I asked myself. The bias of compulsory heterosexuality was in my face. *Was it only cowardice that made her turn toward him,* I wondered, *or was it that she really preferred him to me as a person?*

My feeling was that both Stephane and I liked Eve and were attracted to her, but the heterosexual construction of desire that prevailed in the émigré community made his attraction only acknowledgable. My desire for Eve turned me into the angle of the triangle whose feelings had no words. Biphobia was in action, and I felt bad. At one point Stephane was still living with me and Sara in the compound and spent all his weekends at Eve's. Now the triangulation constructed me as the worn-out "wife" with respect to the newer and more desirable "mistress." I decided I wanted Stephane either completely out of my life or in it for good. So one night I went to Eve's place.

"Why don't you take him in full-time?" I asked her in the kitchen, both of us standing near the table. "He's yours for the taking—I won't reclaim him."

"With my career plan I cannot commit to a relationship," she replied.

"I liked you and I hoped you'd like me. Why did you choose him?"

Eve looked at me flustered and said, "We're all straight here. I don't understand."

"Are you sure? Would you have liked him if he hadn't had me?"

"I am sorry," Eve said as she tuned her eyes away. "I'll take myself out of the situation right away."

I pined from the wounds the game Steal the Phallus was inflicting on me and those I loved. Eve's bisexual panic was a mirror of my anxiety about the triangle's bisexual energy. I did take Stephane back, but my inner voice told me I'd eventually let go of him as well. This triangulation at the center of the émigré community brought my awareness on the energy field between two women involved with the same man. What if the triangle became complete? What if the two women started to love each other as well? Stephane's affair with Eve happened while he was replacing me as a parent during my first career break. Monogamy had been depleting our dual relationship of vital energy, with Sara and Eve functioning as stabilizing forces, third poles in the natural triangulations. They were the vehicles through which the energy between the two of us flowed again. But we were all still hooked on monogamy, which made the crossfire a dangerous place. I lost both Stephane and Eve, and they lost each other as well. My frustration was a call for action to find a bisexual community and embark in the experience of being bi and poly in an open, honest way.

Stephane and I never agreed on what sexual orientation was, but our relationship carried us through a successful completion of our graduate work. Our union came to a crisis in 1985-1986, when, close to graduation, we were groping for a direction which allowed us to stay together while we moved on. It was a long drawn-out battle in which our priorities progressively diverged. He had more power on the job market for, as the favorite male student of a widely known male professor, he was automatically cast as an insider of the ho(m)mosexual confederacy that controls the production of knowledge. He was going to have professional opportunities in America, Europe, and the third world. I was prepared to either be a "permanent temporary" in the United States or an accompanying spouse in the third world, in which both cases I'd follow him into his first employment. There, I would either take advantage of the "sweetheart job" system typical of the United States to get some university teaching employment, or I would bask in the relative largesse in compensating European scientists in the ex-colonies, and devote my energies to my passion for painting.

I was not prepared to follow him to some European country where my paycheck would be necessary to pay the rent but, as the accompanying spouse of a male professor, I would be automatically excluded from the academic career. I also felt that if his commitment to our relationship was serious, there would be a space for my daughter in our plans. Sara was a second grader fluent in English and Italian. She could have gotten an American education either in the United States or in the third world, or an Italian education in Italy, since there is hardly any Italian school abroad. However, I felt that adapting to an educational system in another European language would have not been beneficial to her. It turned out the three of us went our separate ways, which caused a major crisis in my personal life and physical health, a crisis that came at a time when the AIDS crisis was hitting home. Sara went home to Giulio, her dad, and became a little Italian girl. Stephane went to German Switzerland where he met his wife-to-be. And I went to Normal, Illinois, to teach French.

Looking at this time of strife in retrospect, I realize that yes, our power struggles were caused by a sex-gender system that deluded us with a pretense of equality which was not really there, nor were we capable of really envisaging it at all. The fact that neither one of us was a U.S. citizen had its part as well, for we could not help each other get a green card through marriage. I protected my freedom and made the decision I thought was best for Sara and myself. There was something ominous in the project of becoming American, and, as I embarked on it alone, I had no sense of what it would take from me and how deeply I would be transformed in the process. Ultimately, I feel that the intrinsic reason my relationship with Stephane ended is that I needed a source of energy to nurture my English narrative voice into being, and he could neither provide this source nor arrange for our relationship to continue and not be in its way.

III
Hypoglycemia

With Sara back to Italy and her dad, with Stephane off to his first postdoctoral job in Zurich, Switzerland, I was left to face my American destiny alone. The transition between a European-Italian and an Italian-American identity woke me up from the American dream that had taken hold of my imagination, to gradually move toward a planetary feminist ecological consciousness. It implied an appropriation through which, by constructing Sara as part of the female genealogy I claimed for myself, I was reclaiming my own feminist identity. Of course, this identity was still all about independence, and did not yet point to the cosmic interdependence in which all entities share, according to a more planetary ecological consciousness. The academic system instilled its dream of professional success in the only way it could understand it, which was phallic and self-centered. As I woke up I realized I had lost my own dream a long time before—the desire for a more authentic life, one closer to the freedom of nature, that in 1981 had guided me to the Californian shores in the first place. I remember the recurring thought of regretting that Sara had not been named Delia, like my mother. The feminist consciousness I developed during this period was feminine, but it still was a reaction to modernity because it was a reappropriation of what patriarchal culture stole from mothers, rather than a deliverance toward immersion into the body of a living earth.

When I left Italy in 1981, my flight from Sara's father had been a flight from the concept of paternity, and the patriarchal order it engendered. It had been also a response to the normative alcoholism that in modern Italian families served to drown the loss of connection from the energy of mother earth. As a sober person, I was, even at that time, obscurely aware of the effects of drinking on the emotions. I knew that alcohol drowned emotions and made them inexpressible, thus accompanying conventional male personality developments. In the logic of my father and my not-quite-ex-husband, alcohol was a problem only if one drank alone, which, coincidentally, was typical of female alcoholics, for a woman's drinking wasn't socially acceptable. For men, drinking during meals was a natural way to be jovial and sociable, even as the food was more of an excuse than anything else. Desirable women were supposed to enjoy men's joviality, and accompany the drinking in some more moderate way. Censors were left out of the game. I remember my distaste for the wine mixed with water poured to me at banquets when I was seven or eight years old, with the encouragement to savor and get used to it so as to be "a woman of the world." My mother, Delia, was a complete teetotaler, and I turned out to almost be one as well.

As the daughter of a teetotaler who had spent her life in a culture where moderate alcoholism was the norm, I was, even as early as the time when I first I embarked on my immigration process, especially alert to the emotional abuse caused by this problem, and its effect on sober women's health, such as Delia's. I knew how it masked the messages of the body and caused healthy erotic energy to expend itself. Alcoholism was thus the remote-control cause of my parthenogenetic dream of running away from Sara's father, a dream that denied paternity and crumbled when, in 1988, Sara turned me down to stay with Giulio in Rome. Of course, the modern feminist myth of independence was behind my dream as well. In my dreams, I wanted to be the only parent. I wanted to parent and provide as well, so as to demonstrate to the men in my family how unnecessary they were—sperm donors in a female utopia.

During the years 1986 to 1992-1993, I also crossed the boundaries between sexual orientations, first mentally, then emotionally, then physically, and finally in a more spiritual way. These multiple transitions went hand in hand, and their similarity was based on their being structured as processes of inversion, based on an order I believed to be natural which turned out to be cultural instead. The agency of this transition invested several energy fields and included several forces. One was my transformation from a motherly parent, to a distant, often absent parent, one that society automatically constructed as "male." A second area was the progressive distancing between Stephane and myself, which for me implied an estrangement from heterosexuality, a separation between the worlds our union had brought together. A third area was the rearrangement of my inner landscape, including its discursive and linguistic organization. With my dissertation in 1987, I had adopted English as the language of my writing, which implied I had to turn my native languages, both Italian and French, into subsidiary modes of expression that stayed alive under the surface. This implied leaving the island of known emotions to embark in a wide ocean, destination unknown. A fourth area was that of exposing myself to the discriminations inherent to multicultural societies of the first world, where diversity is accepted as long as people are willing to turn themselves into marketable commodities. In this context, marketing is the universal activity in which all players engage, as a tantalizing profusion of merchandises often replaces one's sense of wholeness and self-respect.

Our last year in Riverside together was 1985-1986, and Stephane and I resorted to the free-of-charge therapy services offered by the university's health center, in an effort to sort out the problems in our relationship. He said the system paid for therapy for it knew it could easily drive people crazy. In my optimism, I had not marked this point. He agreed to come on my request, and it was actually during this therapy that he confessed to his affair with Eve.

"She was there when I was alone with your baby in a foreign land. Sara got the flu and the doctor wouldn't even see her without written permission from a biological parent. Eve's presence eased the tension, and we got a bit too close."

What could I say? We patched up our relationship, and, in the fall of 1985, with Sara gone to Italy, we left the family-student compound to reconvene in an off-campus Victorian home shared with three roommates: a graduate student in French and his Californian girlfriend, and a biologist from Montreal, Canada. I must have at least briefly believed it would work, for I remember a passionate French kiss Stephane and I exchanged on a campus bench near the registrar's. The willow shade was pale in the off-white, smoggy air, and we had just turned in our last tuition waivers. Stephane's fleshy lips were soft and mellow, the sweet saliva back and forth between our lips. His tongue, made soft, entered my mouth and touched my teeth and palate. I pushed my tongue into his mouth to get more of that sweet, familiar taste. Both of us had passed our prelims and, no longer afraid of taboos against student-teacher relationships, were ready to express our love on university soil.

It was the fall of 1985 and I had a fellowship to write my dissertation, but I did not write a word because, with Sara gone, I fell in the throes of deep depression. I had wanted this realization of my aspirations to being single and free again, but no, all I could feel was a sense of loss, and every morning when I got up I would just cry and feel bereft, after which I would occupy my day in some low-key effort, desperate that my dissertation project slipped away. The most I could do was read, think, or participate in some cultural event.

Our separate bedrooms were on the first floor, each with a bed and a desk, mine also a walk-in closet. The sash windows looked onto the dusty willows across the road, wrapped in smog. The scruffy wooden floors squeaked under our steps. Spring came, and Stephane was completely absorbed in his experiments. I remember the anxiety of his dissertation, which was based on an elaborate lab experiment that was still not finished two weeks before the closing date. Both of us were under much pressure. As foreigners, we'd be charged nonresident tuition if our graduation was delayed. Our student visas would expire, at which point we'd become deportable and would have to go home with empty hands. Our agreement was that he would finish first and find a job in a city where the three of us would get together again. Since for my dissertation I did not need a laboratory, I would follow and finish there. The tension mounted to a point that was, for me, unbearable. I felt Stephane had a way to leave things for the last minute just to call attention to himself and drive those around him crazy. I was a smoker and, for the first time in my life, my workspace was my bedroom. The ashtray filled up with cigarette butts day after day of nonwork. At night the room was thick with smoke, and I slept in it, which made me feel even more noxious.

One day Stephane and I drove to the nearest harbor to have his personal belongings crated and shipped to France. His dissertation wasn't quite done yet, but time was short. Of course, after that there would be no return on his decision to go back. Not so for me. The doubt started to creep into my consciousness—would I ever return? Europe was saturated with nonpedigreed would-be humanists and intellectuals, who were looked upon as stray dogs, for they were neither ivy-league alumni nor disciples of famous professors. If I went back I'd be one of them, which I thought made my ideas freer and more effective, but wouldn't help when looking for work. I was well aware of how things worked. Even in the best case scenario that, after joining Stephane in his next job, I'd manage to finish my dissertation, all my efforts would not land me the employment I sought. They'd simply prepare me to be a better spouse of a career-oriented male and mother of his kids. True, it was going to be Switzerland and then most likely France, rather than the Italy I came from, but to be honest I did not see that as an improvement.

As we got closer to the harbor, I kept wondering why he was going away. *Why didn't you decide that my professional future is important also? That the best compromise for all three of us is that you stay in the United States?* were my silent questions. He did have a powerful mentor, since the professor with whom he was going to graduate was very well-known and would soon move to Berkeley. I felt left behind, abandoned to my destiny even as we had embarked in our PhD projects counting on mutual support. Yet I longed to be free of him in some way. Part of me never wanted to be a pawn in the game of knowledge as it plays out in high-powered institutions where pure theory is the name of the game. My freedom was too precious, and, even though I was good in theory, I felt theory per se was just a way to keep one's good position in the power game. It skirted the moral imperative of dealing with the political issues at stake. "An elegant scam," I used to think to myself, and argue with Stephane. We must have been in the middle of one of those arguments when, while on the freeway, I enjoined him to let me off. "I would rather hitchhike home than sit next to you one more minute," I said. I was sick and he wouldn't listen.

"Don't be so nervous, Gaia," he said as he kept driving. "I'm returning home, and will spend two weeks with my parents in Southern

France. Then I will start my new job in Zurich, Switzerland. When you're ready, you're welcome to join me."

I kept wondering, how would it feel to be his companion and would-be spouse in France, me, a foreign woman with a foreign daughter from another man? Liberal as France had been historically, including as a host to Italian expatriates during the Fascist *ventennio,* I imagined it would not welcome me, nor would it encourage my professional aspirations.

While I was taking my distance from Stephane and our relationship, I also gradually lost my health and physical energy. I developed what appeared to be an emotional disorder, which made my moods swing from grandly euphoric to deeply depressed, and put me at risk for suicide at every turn. I remember driving the old Plymouth Duster in downtown Riverside, in the middle of the thickest smog. The desire to kill myself would surge prominently, as a tree appeared on the side of the road, and I'd want to drive right into it. Sometimes it was a car coming in the opposite direction, and I had to make a major effort to keep my mind focused on the fact that I would also most likely kill another person. I realized I was dangerous and asked for help, which I got from our roommate Michel. I had always had a sweet tooth, and this tendency became more prominent as I felt abandoned and unprepared to manage my situation. There were only a few days before Stephane's dissertation was due; his flight was scheduled. We were friends with a couple from Italy, Paola, a biologist, and Pietro, an architect. Their first cousins ran the classiest Italian restaurant in LA, the Rex, and had a wonderful home whose fridge was full of the most delicious day-old desserts. They suggested I stay there for a few days, just to get away from the stress of it all. My sweet tooth betrayed me and I pigged out on those desserts, which only made things worse. When I returned to Riverside I went to the student health center and insisted on an urgent appointment with a psychiatrist from the nearby mental hospital, in Loma Linda. Sure enough, Stephane's dire predictions were coming true—the system had driven me crazy and it was time to get ready for the loony asylum, which would confirm that I had never been PhD material in the first place.

Well, Paola, the female biologist from Italy, rescued me. "You have strange reactions to food," she observed one day as we had dinner with her, "especially sweets. You might have an imbalance of glucose in your blood, just like a diabetic or hypoglycemic person. I think you should get your glucose level tested."

I returned to the center where they were reluctant to test me. I told them I'd not budge until a test was scheduled. I did test positive for this dangerous nutritional imbalance, which, accidentally, as I was told, caused Virginia Woolf's suicide. Hypoglycemia is a syndrome few conventional doctors understand. It is a prelude to diabetes, as well as its opposite, since the production of insulin is accelerated. A naturopath was called, and he told me what I had, explaining how the condition had to be brought under control by an appropriate diet and eating style. Meals had to be frequent and small; their staple complex carbohydrates, such as whole-food grains, fibers, and cereals, which gradually release energy into the blood, thus keeping one's glucose level in balance and one's moods stable. Raw fruits and vegetables were the complement. Also, of course, no sweets, alcohol, coffee, or smoking. This naturopath and Paola, the Italian biologist, believed that my mind still worked and saved me from the loony asylum and antidepressants. They set me on the path that would lead me, years later, to embrace my vegetarian tendencies, which became more acceptable as the holistic health movement became more popular.

As a result of this diagnosis I quit smoking. It was during my summer trip to visit Italy and my family, and I remember making the decision one night in Rome while having dinner with my brother, Andrea, and our father, who quit in his late forties after our mother's death from cancer. Andrea, who was now living in England, announced he had just quit, and I thought I must do the same. *You want to last as long as he does, don't you?* I told myself. So I quit cold turkey, and never started again. Back in Riverside in the fall, the UCR library offered me a carrel, a small private room to write and keep my work in progress. Ivy leaves climbed alongside the carrel window. The air was still and transparent; the world outside just a remote buzz with its worries and preoccupations—books all around me, their smell of mystery and incantation. As I entered the space, I realized it was there that I was going to write my dissertation. Now I was a nonsmoker and I belonged. I wrote Stephane a letter, that I had found the place, would he please wait until I was done also? Maybe I had changed my mind about joining him, but we'd leave the details for later. I was confident he would accept. He was a major meat eater, and, like most French people, had his steak a bleeding rare, which I found unseemly. Both of us were participants in cultures famous for their elaborate cuisine, and so together we would tend to eat gourmet rather than healthy. But now I knew that food had an effect on my mental energy, and felt that a complete control over my diet was the only way to recover my health. I was prepared to live alone if necessary, and explained why. And so the job was undertaken, and my dissertation started to pour out of me in those long hours in the carrel. Having followed the doctor's advice for the most part—except for coffee, which I quit many years later—my condition did not develop into diabetes, and in a few years I was in full recovery, having benefited from the following measures: living alone so as to be able to fully control my time, space, sleep, and food intake; quitting smoking; and keeping no sweets at home.

But there were things I did not understand, and it was going to take much longer for me to get there. This illness of mine was not taken seriously by the people I knew because they had not even heard of it. It is the kind of ailment that Western medicine does not understand, and it is often not diagnosed until it has actually turned into diabetes or neurosis. On the other hand, my folks had always thought I was kind of nuts in a way. My "folks" now of course were my father, Dario, and his second wife, Marina. They were really not part of my life in the United States, and I remember that I rarely mentioned the fact that I was, in some way, a red-diaper baby, for my father's career in politics was in the Italian Communist Party, even though as an independent. For most of her life Marina had been a secretary, and she seemed to think of that as a most appropriate woman's job. Dario, of course, did not argue with her. So, all the aspirations that my mother had for me were kind of dead, buried under the memory of the illness that took her away. True, Marina was an American citizen. A war bride who ran away with a G.I. at the end of World War II, she had married a foreigner, divorced him, and returned. Surely she knew about defiance and transgression. But she seemed to feel that all my attempts to imitate this side of her were wrong. Hadn't I gotten out of an all right marriage in a somewhat unjustified way? Hadn't I had the presumption to think that, as a single woman, I could just take off and create a life for myself in America? And what about my wanting to study all these literary things, wasn't that kind of nutty and useless anyway? Under the pragmatic influence of Marina and my grandmother Teresa before her, literature, philosophy, and artistic expression were useless and impracticable aspirations, especially for a girl. They were a sign of madness, and my physical symptoms, a difficulty in communicating, moments of terrible weakness and depression, dizzy spells, inexplicable longings that neither I nor they could understand, would only confirm their conjecture. Women's health was a problem in the family, and I had sort of completed my reproductive job already. Had they known about my condition, I bet they would have put me away and visited me on Sundays to tell me all about their successes. Wasn't that what they did at my mother's grave?

With these questions in mind, I was finishing my dissertation. I kept my focus on the memory of Delia, who had visited me a year earlier, while Stephane and Eve were having the affair. It was 1984 and I was in the train from Rome to Florence. I had an appointment with Franca Rame, the wife of a famous playwright, Dario Fo. I wanted to interview her as part of my dissertation research, for I suspected Franca contributed to his work. The compartment was empty as the train entered a long tunnel. Delia's body felt vividly present, with her voice and breath. She said, "This is what you were meant to do. This is your purpose." I was a bit surprised for I didn't believe in ghosts. *It must be a hallucination,* I thought, but it was inspiring and I followed.

Now in 1986, Stephane, in Zurich, was still confident I'd finish and join him. But in the Old World the couple was not an institution as sacred as it is in the United States. There would be no "sweetheart jobs." I wondered, *Why finish if it is to blend my life to his and live in the shadow of his profession? Do I need my PhD for him to like me? For me to like myself? If I do finish my PhD, maybe I won't follow him, for I will want a career of my own. How come he does not consider following me instead?*

Initially, my dissertation included a discussion of *The Children's Hour,* a play in which a woman falls in love with another woman. But eventually, I edited out that section. *Maybe it will give away my secret and the committee won't let me graduate.* For them I already was a single mother and a foreigner. *Let's not confuse them too much or they won't let me graduate.* This play marked my acknowledgment of my bisexuality and anticipated the erotic dream of a threesome with both Stephane and his Swiss girlfriend that helped me forgive them. I now realize that Eve, like me, only wanted to be part of the game. But compersion, or the joy of seeing one's partner enjoy erotic love with another person, was not a known feeling to me yet.

IV
Parthenogenesis

It was the fall of 1987 and I had moved to Illinois for my first job in Normal, at Illinois State University. The town was just as plain as its name and it was surrounded with oceanic cornfields open to the winds of the Mississippi basin. The streets formed a regular grid, and were lined with two-story homes, regularly spaced and topped with slanted gray roofs looking up toward maple-tree branches.

My relationship with Stephane had turned transcontinental, which brought devastating developments. E-mail was not common yet, and our long-distance communication was based on long phone calls and infrequent visits. My body ached. I was used to that constant presence, that daily interaction—I could not function alone. We met several times for a few days in various neutral locations along the trajectory between our separate stations.

Stephane was relearning to be European, with the small spaces, the formalisms, the claustrophobia that lifestyle involved. I was curious about that, but not persuaded I wanted it for myself. In my New-World life, I was an immigrant and so I was alone—wondering why nobody joined me. I did not have the stability to form another heterosexual relationship, but did get signs of interest from lesbians. Indeed, Stephane and I noticed that on our own, both of us got sexual attention from gays. We found it exciting and scary. There was more transience in that world, sexual players didn't mind that one might soon be gone. It was the early AIDS scare, with its eerie tales of infection. We were thrilled about our new sexual discoveries, but afraid they'd drive us further apart.

That long 1987-1988 winter in Illinois was a period of incredible loneliness for me. The sleeping around, the casual sex, the improvised communions between souls that, before Stephane, had provided access to the sacred for me, were over. We knew very little about safer sex and were not sure what sexual behaviors were risky and how the risk could be offset. We didn't know exactly what to be afraid of. I remember once at an overseas conference in West Berlin, the typical place where one would for sure get laid, having played the game as usual, and having found the right guy to take to my bedroom. And then, the paralysis: was kissing okay? How do you get your juices going if you can't even touch the other person? Yes, our condoms were ready, but how do you get there when body fluids can't be exchanged? It was the first time that I felt powerless in the game of sex. I compared myself to those people who are rendered frigid by religious upbringing or repressive education. The paralysis ended in a nonevent, which threw me into one of the worst hypoglycemia crises I ever had. The guy was gone, and the next day I found myself unable to get out of bed. I was all alone, since Geraldine, who had come to Berlin to visit me from Geneva, had already left. I was scheduled to be on a plane and could not get out of bed. The next day, when I finally felt a little better, I went to the airport anyway, and for some reason nobody noticed that I had a closed ticket and was scheduled to travel the day before. I promised myself never to leave home again without a small supply of transportable complex carbohydrates. As I got home to Normal, I stuffed granola bars everywhere, in the glove compartment, in my purse, in the office, in my suitcases, and regarded these small packets as my lifeline for years to come.

It was also a time of reflection, from a distance, about the management of Sara's biculturalism, and the way things would pan out if she returned to the United States. While still in Riverside, in the summer when school let out, the three of us used to take a short vacation, visiting the national parks of the western region, the Grand Canyon, Yosemite, Mesa Verde, the Mojave Desert, and other areas where one got a sense of Gaia, the Earth, as a living organism. Stephane was a great guide, since he knew about soil science and geology. Sara loved it, but of course our hikes presumed a certain fitness and physical strength. After these trips she would spend the summer in Sardinia with her grandparents on Giulio's side, while he was also there on vacation. Sara was the only messenger between the two worlds she inhabited, and this was far from being easy on both of us and her. It must have been a challenge to her grandparents as well. Whenever she came back Stephane and I found out that her vision of her experience had changed. Obviously, her grandparents asked about her life in the United States, and of course she told them. But to them those adventures must have seemed enormously strange and perilous. "The Grand Canyon, cowboys, guns, Indians, as in a picture starring John Wayne." Surely, she was not being raised to become a docile, god-fearing female, "what would eventually become of her?" There was even more bewilderment about food. When Sara was with us she ate everything we ate. There were no favoritisms and no capricious behavior. But with her grandmother, she was the one who dictated the menu, which is typical of overprotective Italian grandparents. "I don't want spinach, *Nonna*. Make me some soup instead," she'd order. So, on her return she refused what we served at our table, even though that food had been so dearly earned for her.

She did not pass judgment on our lifestyle or object to the relationship Stephane and I had, but in a way, judgment was passed through her, for her effort to unify her worlds made the different points of view transparent. I wished I could protect our nuclear family from the influence of traditionalist grandparents as my mother did with hers. But I was a student and needed the help, for the summer months were a time to prepare for upcoming courses and seminars, as well as prelims and other major exams. We were doing the right thing, we were getting an education, the best we could afford. But a sense of illegitimacy surrounded our relationship, as a union between foreigners, neither sanctified nor blessed.

I felt I'd never be able to find myself as long as Sara moved back and forth. I wanted to become her only parent, and only a good academic job would have made that possible. I felt somebody from afar watching my every motion, and doing it through the person I loved most. When the decision to send Sara back to Giulio was made, I did not really oppose it. I felt it was time he became more responsible, instead of having his parents do his job. I could not get Giulio to support Sara while I raised her, and I forced him to raise her instead. But when the pain of having lost her came, I did not hesitate to blame Stephane for insisting on sending her away. I was not aware of how my own internalized biphobia, and my desire to explore what it meant, might have precipitated my decision as well.

This blame, deserved or not, made me unable to love Stephane anymore. The mere sight of him reminded me of Sara and this made the pain of having lost her more unbearable. I wished humans had parthenogenesis like cells, that each of us could have a kid without any genetic input from the outside. So on the one hand I participated in the decision that would make Sara more Italian, on the other I set out on a path that gratified my desire to explore forms of erotic expression beyond heterosexual monogamy. I wasn't sure Stephane would follow me, but it was important to try. At one point I had desired a child from Stephane. But at this time the last thing I wanted was another "husband" and baby who would then tie me up in another no-exit relationship. What with being a single mother of two, with two very different exes, their respective families, and their impossible-to-meet demands? The least I could do, I thought, was spare Sara the risk of having a brother, and being relegated to the frustrating position I had in my family, as the oldest child and a girl followed by a boy. I vowed to put my professional training to use and ensure a future better than mine for her.

Part of the reason for shipping Sara off was precisely my fear that Stephane and I would not work out an arrangement, and I'd end up on my own. Then I'd live in a country where I could not legally work, while being financially responsible for both Sara and myself. This would make it impossible for me to turn myself into a job-market commodity able to get the high-profile academic employment that would grant my green card and right to work. I wanted my PhD to offer Sara a better future. However, paradoxically, keeping her with me at that time meant throwing the market value of my degree away. The situation was just too risky and unstable for her. Many times later I told myself that I should have asked Giulio to send me money for her, that I should have insisted on keeping Sara with me, and that perhaps the support I needed would have materialized if I had only believed I could get it. But I felt responsible for abandoning the men in my life, my father, and Giulio, my not-quite-ex, and did not realize they failed to support me in my endeavors, even as my body told me their abusive manners had to be fled.

Part of me wanted my daughter to grow up Italian. I wanted her to have the privilege of growing up in a space where she was not an ethnic type or a foreigner, where the faces of the people around her would mirror her own. But at the time I was not sure because the languages of my subconscious did not get along. My professors explained that for Lacan, language is shaped like the subconscious. Lacan, of course, was French, and he spoke and thought in that language. But what happens, I asked myself, when a person's experience registers and is acted out in several languages? Does the subconscious become fragmented? Does it multiply? I am not sure but at that time I felt I had three subconscious voices, one French, one English, and one Italian. Each one gave me orders that conflicted with the other two. Part of me must have been leery of saddling Sara with a similar torment. The only times I had been happy as a parent were in our family student compound where Sara ran around in the street all day, with her multiracial playmates. At home in the compound, we applied my mother's clothing-optional policies, used three languages, and ate, spoke, and behaved in multicultural ways. But her dad and his family also had something to offer her, which could not reach her in the United States. It was a sense of rootedness, of ancestry, of knowing the mountains, the trees, the animals, the stones, the plants that were part of one's surroundings. Being present to the landscape for generations, and inheriting a language that reflected that presence, was a legacy she could only get from the premodern side of her family. Her Sardinian relatives were part of that old-world ecology I missed in the "New World."

Not that I didn't feel responsible for sending my little girl back to a man I had kicked out of my life partly on account of alcohol. My decision was in some ways sustained by the wish that he would do for her what he'd not done for me, reform and be a good parent. Ironically, sending Sara to him seemed the only way to realize my dream of a world where I'd be the only parent. Eventually, I thought, my higher job-market value would make Giulio unnecessary, and I'd become the only source of emotional and material care. Of course, I did not realize how offensive my parthenogenetic fantasy was. But foisting Sara on Giulio resulted in a very positive relationship between them, which I sometimes came to resent. Eventually, my parthenogenetic dream dissolved into a more holistic dream, based on feminist ecology and a vision of shared, communal parenting.

When the separation between Stephane and I happened, I felt the relationship had run its course. The contents of our inner landscapes had transmigrated from his to mine and vice versa. His knowledge of scientific and environmental problems had found its way into my consciousness more than I was aware of. Like a good child of artist parents, Stephane was completely subject to my gaze, he was used to being looked at as a painter's model and derived a subdued pleasure from it. This subjection gave me a measure of my own talent and power to express it. Much as he hated it, he was the perfect model, and I adored the passivity that entailed. As for many scientists, his knowledge of any language was basic, yet he was very familiar with the sense of Italian culture I inherited from my parents, including literature and politics. I thought of his childhood memories of canned raviolis, and of Sara's lesson on rolling spaghettis on her arrival in 1982. It was now four years later, and the two of us walked alongside a good-looking but not very high-quality Italian restaurant in Santa Monica one day. He casually glanced at the spaghettis that one of the customers held on his fork, then turned to me with a semi-disgusted expression and said, "That pasta doesn't look very al dente, does it?" Even from a distance, he could estimate the extent to which the spaghettis served on that plate were overcooked. He had hybridized quite a lot and shared a body of knowledge with us. These structures of feeling had entered his consciousness through our mutual acquaintance and frequentation. And precisely because I felt that a substantial part of this transmigration had happened already, I approved of our decision to part ways. I knew this decision came at the right moment, even though, at the time, it was difficult to metabolize and fraught with the unknown challenges that lay ahead.

V
Empty Forms

The Midwest was to remain foreign to me, for I had a two-semester appointment there, from the fall of 1987 to the spring of 1988, and my spirit was in such turmoil that I could barely notice what surrounded me. But I do remember the town, Normal, and my apartment. I decorated the living room with a Mexican hammock whose shades of green and orange contrasted with the light gray color of the sky. The bedroom window looked upon a small yard with a large maple tree. In the fall, I watched the leaves change colors every day, from spots of light yellow spreading through the green mass, to the shades of brown and red as the cold was drying them, to the dark outline of the naked branches against the sky. The whole process was amplified with respect to more temperate climates. I must have looked unprepared for the winter, for a colleague from Lebanon who had lived in Chicago for twelve years kept bringing her hand-me-down coats, mittens, and gloves to my place. She was worried. "Never leave the apartment without them," she urged. The advent of spring was as magnified as the other season changes, as the smells of blossoms flew North through the wide Mississippi Valley, and the wind announced the new season at least two weeks ahead. I had never seen a natural phenomenon of such wide proportions, an ecosystem of such vastness. I looked at the landscape and it was just as bare as in the winter months, but its fragrance betrayed the secret of its soon-to-be-sprouting plants. I tried to adapt the language of my native Mediterranean ecology, with its tiny ecosystems and swift transitional seasons, to the present circumstances. I imagined Botticelli's Primavera as a large, veiled fairy hiding in a cloud, whose transparent mantle sprinkled the valley with invisible fresh buds.

I was finally making a decent living and decided to have my paintings framed and shown at a café in nearby Champaign-Urbana. But

Stephane had been the model for most of them, and so the wound oozed. My Lebanese colleague and I used to drive to Champaign for a chocolate mousse at Timpone's. It was the only diversion available, until, to our great surprise, a local café opened up. For the sixty miles covered, the road was completely flat. I had never seen such a plain and was in awe of its proportions. My colleague advised that it could be deadly in a snowstorm. "Keep blankets and candles in your trunk," she recommended. But as harvest time approached, the soil turned into an expanse of blond spikes waving in the sun.

During this first period as a single person, the myth of modernity co-opted me completely and relentlessly. I was being sucked into the materialistic, acquisitive philosophy of industrial development. There were no residues, no memory of old-world ecologies, no remnants of more sustainable lifestyles. Ironically, this was also the time when my desire to escape to the third world was most intense. Having no access of my own to that cultural space, I still unrealistically counted on Stephane's agricultural expertise. The possibility of continuing our relationship was still open as neither one of us was settled in our respective jobs. During my year in the Midwest, in September, I received a call that he was invited at the institute for agricultural studies in Los Baños, near Manila, Philippines. While still in Riverside, we had discussed the possibility of going there already, along with another institute in Ibadan, near Lagos, Nigeria. To me these seemed much sunnier and happier options than making his return to Europe final, especially if Europe meant a North European country with little sunshine and frozen souls, where his companion would have to take a day job just to carry her weight. To me, at least, the agricultural institutes in these third-world locations had so much more to offer: Sara would enroll in an American or British school located near them, and I would not have to work for money, which would mean I could devote myself to developing my artistic talent. And there would be so many beautiful and exotic and colorful things to paint! When we were still together, I used to tease Stephane that I found black men very attractive. I think he imagined that once in Africa, I'd fall in bed with a couple of them.

Both of us were aware of the ambiguous position of Western scientists in the third world, as representatives of an order that caused maldevelopment in the first place. But neither could anticipate that at Cold War's end, the situation of these countries would get worse. Yet freedom from economic necessity was not the only thing that attracted me to that choice. There was also a sense of gravity, a feeling of wanting to be down there, where life is a gift and is not taken for granted, where one's environment has not been transformed in a profusion of merchandises, and being relates to body in a more intense way. But Stephane did not see it that way. Europe seemed to him a primary status goal, and he felt that indulging one's time in the third world would make a comeback more difficult, if not impossible. I tend to think that to these rather stodgy considerations one must add the fact that his parents were very old, and that he felt the responsibility of being near them when their lives would come to an end.

I remember that a few days after my thirty-third birthday, Stephane called to tell me that he had been offered the Manila job. I said, "If you accept it, I will follow you at the end of the school year."

"But the boss there thinks that European women don't adjust easily to life at the base," he objected. "He says I should go alone and find a woman there."

"Which European women is your boss talking about? I grew up at the border of the third world, since Southern Italy is often considered part of that area. I have adjusted to Southern California already, which was a whole other ball game. What makes you think I wouldn't adjust to the Philippines? Perhaps your German Swiss girlfriend won't, but I would—I'm sure you know."

The conversation ended on this note, and I knew he was going to turn down the offer and stay with his European mate. A few days later I received a carved-wood mask from the Philippines, which is now part of my collection and still hangs from my living room wall. The same week a fat letter from him arrived, and I opened it with trepidation, only to discover that it was my letter he had sent back to me—the one in which in an excess of pathos, I had confessed to him that I wished Sara had never been born, so that I could have been free to follow him anywhere. The letter also said that I had kept no copy, which was a way to tell him "it's for you, not for posterity; it's how I feel, not a writer's trick," since I knew he felt manipulated by my aspirations for artistic and literary expression. A note on it said, "This letter is really very beautiful, but you must forget me."

I felt bereft. Geraldine was the only person still connected to both Stephane and myself. "Our relationship is falling apart," I explained to her on the phone. "I want to go with him to Manila and he wants to stay in Switzerland and marry his new girlfriend. I am here all alone in Illinois with these devastating phone calls."

Suddenly, I realize my female friend is more important than my male lovers. "Maybe there's a mistake," I tell her. "We should try something different between ourselves."

But Geraldine is not open. "I tried once," she says, "I could not touch her. The female body horrifies me."

Next time, I think. *Wrong person, not yet.*

As I got accustomed to my wished-for single status, I also learned that to satisfy my sexual yearnings I often had to count primarily on myself. Even with all the liberalism with respect to the body of my childhood household, I had never learned or practiced the art of self-pleasuring. My mother, who, even in her short-shrift life, had managed to explain everything about intercourse, fertilization, and childbirth, never quite got to masturbation. In my peer culture as an adolescent, self-pleasuring was perceived as a cop-out, a cowardly withdrawal from more intersubjective ways of sexual expression. It was in no way perceived as a brave way to come to a better knowledge of oneself. I always had male partners, which taught me how to derive my own pleasure from their bodies, rather than from my own. Now I was faced with the fact that if I wanted balance and a sense of self-centeredness, I had to learn how to deal with my yearnings on my own. I knew this would enhance the exchange of pleasure in new partner-based sexual relationships. But the body of my French lover was so ingrained in my imagination that for the first two years it was the only fantasy ever present to me.

Heterosexuality was becoming an empty form. When Stephane's choices turned my most egalitarian relationship into a power game, I began to see it as a marker of status and success. I did not really mind that another woman had been chosen, one more docile and submissive than I was. But I could not have been fully aware of the extent to which my profession was now all I had left and could count on, with all the risks thereof. As a foreigner, I knew I needed a tenure-track appointment to get my labor certification. As a woman, I knew that my gender would play in my favor if the equal opportunities opened by Affirmative Action came my way. Luckily, the English Department at Lovelace University, in Netherville, Tennessee, had invited me on campus for an interview. I checked out the books published by its professors for I wanted to know what was in their heads. I knew how useful this knowledge could be in the interviewing process. I found some of the books quite interesting and imagined their authors as I read them. I would have liked to return to California, but I knew there were no options for foreign PhDs there, for the naturalization process was clogged up by immigrants from nearby Mexico and central America. On top of that, institutions were busy hiring people from local minorities to comply with affirmative action regulations. I knew of a colleague at Riverside who was originally a subject of the British Crown, yet his green card had arrived the year he made tenure, which doubled the agony of the seven-year probation period, his ageing mother in Wales longing for a visit. But the country's heartland was a different story. Immigration procedures were more expeditious due to a lower flow. Back there, foreigners could be counted as minorities for hiring purposes, but the irony was that in the center of the nation all diverse people were cruelly stigmatized.

The department that invited me had been the birthplace of New Criticism, a school of thought that discouraged the study of literature in its cultural contexts. It was also influenced by the Agrarians, with their aristocratic nostalgia for antebellum society and the institution of slavery. Even though I was not fully aware of my diversities or the perception thereof, I had no doubts that I was going to be diverse enough. I had been warned to avoid them, but I did not really have a choice because my American PhD was useless without U.S. citizenship. I had no relatives in the United States. Fake marriage was not uncommon for noncitizens in my position, but for me it was out of the question for I had never quite divorced Giulio. I went. My genteel hosts put up a façade of civility for my two-day visit and I believed it.

At about the same time, in prissy Netherville, the police were intent in cleaning up the city's sites of public sex by entrapping men who, unaware, accosted fifteen- to seventeen-year-old police decoys. Their voices were taped and even though they hadn't done anything yet, they were arrested after a few days. It was the city's way to process the AIDS scare. A few of the victims were professors, while the police decoys were young enough to be their students. I had an obscure awareness of the fact that a favorite student can offer a teacher a semblance of the self-reflection we often look for in others like ourselves. When I heard the story a year later, the agony of the situation pierced my consciousness, and I learned something about my profession I feel is still true today. *Of course we fall in love with our students. We all do; we have to. What is teaching if not love? Love of the person we see the student become, love of his or her potential, love of what has passed over through the creative and intellectual energy generated in the learning process.*

Back to Italy for the summer break, Stephane's presence became stronger in my inner landscape. From Italy I traveled by train across Europe to meet him in Alsace-Lorraine. He was determined to break up the relationship for he wanted to be with his new girlfriend, who lived in Basel where she had a good job, which was near the European city where he worked, and not across the ocean. Yet he had accepted that the two of us get together for one last time, in a nice, romantic place, to say good-bye in a complete, intense way. I remember my mind thinking, while I was on the train, that when the two of us would get together in the hotel room, I'd play our male-rape game, and stay on top of him until he came, and thus get pregnant. Some Freudian trips played in my head: *You get his baby, you get him.* Not that I was in the mood for raising another child, but I did like his genes, and felt justified by our years together for wanting a little piece to myself. The time was ripe, and, on that train, I felt like an eel swimming upstream to find "fertility paradises," as the Italian poet Eugenio Montale would say.

When in the room, my male-rape trick did work, as it always did, giving me a measure of the power of our teacher-student eros. The grip I had on his body almost scared me, since it must have been similar to the one he had on mine. In some ways this reminded me of Antonio, my father's *padre/maestro,* and the control over Dario's emotions this father/teacher must have had. (Was that the cause of Dario's inclination to create relationships of the totalizing kind—that left no distance between partners and no room for anything else?) Now I was measuring my own mastery. But I pulled off the minute before Stephane came, and went quickly to the bathroom to finish myself. I had to give myself the last stroke to feel like a human being again. I never told him about my plan to get pregnant, yet maybe the same thought crossed his mind also, but this child was never conceived, and we went our separate ways.

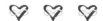

I chose to be the center of my life, not because the other life was not worth following, but because I felt the need to accomplish something with my own. Finishing my dissertation became easy once the choice was made. I was not connected to female sexual energy yet, but I knew that what I knew about sexuality was not enough. I could see the big pretension that heterosexuality was ever since Stephane started to date his Swiss girlfriend. I felt he wanted to prove to me he could replace me. I felt a strong, perverse desire to go there and seduce the other woman, tell her "all Stephane knows about sex he learned from me." I imagined a seduction à la *The Conformist* or *Dangerous Liaisons,* lurking, fearful, dishonest because it was based on hatred and not love. With another woman in the position of Stephane's partner, my return to Europe was no longer an option. I felt betrayed but decided to leave them alone. Horrified by my feelings and depressed about myself, I wished I knew how to connect to female sexual energy in positive ways.

Eventually, Stephane married and had two children and I went on to experience an extended period as a single person. For many years the best expression of friendship Stephane and I could offer each other was no expression at all. Silence was the best way to protect the precarious equilibrium we had managed to create for ourselves as separate persons. It was many years later that the two of us became e-mail friends and resumed our conversations in cyberspace.

VI
MLA

My most acute nomadic phase began in the fall of 1988, when, with my PhD in sight, I transformed myself into a job-market commodity primed and packaged for the shop-windows of the academic conference-and-interviewing circuit. It was forced nomadism, since I was barely aware of what I was getting into. As a good imitator, I did orchestrate a rather successful advertising campaign for myself and passed for a highly desirable candidate. Yet a deep sense of alienation was present in my consciousness. I experienced the job search as a loss of self, and self meant roots, community, and connectedness with the regional culture that had adopted me during my graduate studies, its climate and landscape.

At Riverside, I had been instructed on the academic job market by one of my professors, B. J., who was the most aware of what was going on. His lover Karen, Stephane, he, and I had been good friends, often going on day trips to LA for theater and other, more esoteric and impressive performance-art events, such as those by Judy Chicago and Susan Lacy. They also initiated us to the conventions of the MLA. It was a big conference held in a major U.S. city between Christmas and New Year's, where applicants who had been short-listed for a job would be interviewed. Then, if they became finalists, they would be invited for a campus interview as well, after which the school would make its final choice.

I did not know what a job market was, for Italy never had one. Things were done by family connections and favoritism, as both my brother Andrea and I knew very well, being the children of an independent senator who railed against the system at every turn—thus making enough enemies to drive both of us abroad. I had never seen a system operate in which initiative and merit had a function, and I was thrilled to be now in a place where this happened. I knew I was a hard worker and a capable person, so it all boded very well. I had decent looks and manners, and was confident I would do well.

But there was something bizarre and a bit grotesque to it all. I asked why the conference was such an odd time of year. *Aren't people spending the holidays with their families?* I wondered. Well, as it turned out, this was the only week that all universities were closed and professors were not away on research. I came from an atheist family but was accustomed to spending the holidays in the intimacy of those I knew. It was a time of privacy and reflection, regardless of any religious service. But here conference participants were caught in a whirlwind of frantic activity surrounded by strangers, some of whom would soon have the power of life and death over them.

The MLA was hosted in uncharacteristic luxury chains such as the Marriott and Sheraton. These hotels had no local character; they were just large, glamorous, and anonymous. Participants dressed somewhat formally, three-piece suits for boys, and padded-shoulder jackets with skirts and pumps for girls. But from their movements you could tell they were not used to that kind of attire. It was like a dress-rehearsal performance where you see that costumes have just arrived from the tailor's shop. On top of that, people seemed to have a strange script in their heads, which can be summarized as, "Speak only to those who count or are perceived as such, and treat everybody else as if they were completely transparent." "If in the middle of a conversation, you realize you've mistaken a person who does not count for one who does, drop the conversation immediately and run away." In the elevator people did not say hello, but looked at your badge to measure your worth, based on whether or not they recognized your name and the institution you were from. This was rather embarrassing, for most academics don't have 20/20 vision, and so the way they ignored your face and the courtesy of greeting your presence was self-evident as their eyes squinted at the badge on your chest.

I thought this was a place where members of the same profession came together to get to know one another and feel proud of the community they were part of—a place to feel welcome and welcome others, especially newcomers. But in the hallways, people would stand up and talk to one another surreptitiously and hurridly. If you ap-

proached them, they would not open the circle and let you participate, but would rather look very disturbed, as if you were intruding
on some conspiracy. This was the cultural elite of the nation, and I
thought it was surprising that they seemed to know nothing about
common courtesy. They were more specialized than the professoriat
of any nation, for the system had more room for specialties and more
money for research, yet they seemed to have learned nothing from all
the books they'd read, nor have the slightest sense of manners and
considerate public behavior. As I later learned, that standoffish attitude was due to a general difficulty in communication throughout the
profession, as people just barely had seconds to pass vital pieces of information to their friends, and as this grapevine was better left off the
record to avoid the liabilities it could generate.

But what was most amazing was the way you met your future colleagues, the persons who had the power to both change your life and
enter it in a forceful way. You met them in their bedroom, as they responded to your timid knock on the door that bore the room number
you got from the house phone downstairs. To me, it was surprising
enough that, at that time of year, a convention would not turn into a
party, as it would in many merrier and more festive cultural spaces.
But as décors for a professional conversation, those lavish bedrooms
appeared more suitable for the luxurious movie industry than for the
sterner academic profession.

In the late 1980s, about as many female candidates were on the
market as male, most professors in a position to hire were male, and
academic culture was still heavily heterosexist. Therefore, several in-
terviewers were present on each occasion, which helped to allay possible anxieties related to sexual harassment or the perception thereof.
The sense of intimacy in the situation caused the weaker parties to feel
vulnerable and subject to a closeness that I thought was neither desirable nor necessary. People would get excited and involved in the game
of exchanging gazes. The point of the interview was often lost. Things
never got rough for me; I never felt intentionally harassed nor disres-
pected. But I remember my thoughts during a one-hour conversation
about the theater and its many seductive intricacies with a male inter-
viewer who was alone. We were sitting on opposite armchairs in a

spacious room with dark-green flowered curtains. He was a handsome man in his forties with a good figure, tall, elegant, and with an intellectual flair, his dark hair extending to the nape of his neck. I imagined how it would feel to fuck him on the nearby king-size bed. I am sure it would have been fun, and wonder if the same idea crossed his mind also. It was not one of the interviews that went further, and I have no regrets for I was weary of potential lovers with the power to turn me into their protégée.

I wonder, though, if he was turned on by me, would he have seen me as a sexual peril and not pursued me as a job candidate?

I had interviews with many schools, including Purdue and Cornell, except, of course, the most prestigious Ivy Leagues, who interviewed only among themselves. I was a bit miffed that UCLA or UC Berkeley would not look at good candidates from the UC system at large, except, perhaps, when they desperately needed a minority person, for I felt such practice would only strengthen higher education in their own state. But star wars were in fashion, and academics had learned to play. To affirm its power, an institution had to catch candidates whose stars were flying high, from traditional schools like Harvard and Yale. As the candidate moved to the UC campus that now aspired to Ivy-League status, the prestige of the Eastern Seaboard would transfer from coast to coast. I knew I was not part of this game, since Riverside established its reputation while I was there, and currently had no history of prestige.

The first time around the system had landed me in Normal, where I was suffering from my excruciating romantic pains and the local student population felt so foreign that the cornfields looked to me like a copy of their straight blond hair. How different from the Pasolinian dark curls that encircled the faces of my Roman classmates! Supposedly, we all were of the same race, but these differences had an impact on the way I felt as a teacher in those areas. Much later I became aware of the cruelty of my comparison, when I learned that at harvest time the blond-haired students turned themselves into field workers. For most of them French was a requirement to get over with, and I doubt they could imagine it as a language actually spoken as the primary means of communication in many parts of the world. Of course, the textbook, a remnant of the age that the 1968 revolution has swept away, did not help. I was ashamed to use those stilted sentences that made the language that most aroused my erotic imagination sound dead. But then, of course, suggesting a new textbook would have been completely out of place on my part. I despaired that any of the French I taught would actually get into those students' heads. Yet this cruelty was a mere reflection of the way I felt, in an educational environment so mired in its own parochialism that learning became a purely mechanical process.

But I still managed to play the job-market game, and so, in February 1988, well-packaged as a newly groomed expert, I flew to Tennessee to interview for my first tenure-track job, which could be regarded as the fulfillment of my aspirations. It was a position in drama in a department of English that granted graduate degrees and was part of a well-endowed university. This invitation valued the knowledge I had acquired based on my studies, dedication, and merits. It had nothing to do with the native language skills I share with anybody who grew up in Rome. I had heard negative tales about the South and the way foreigners were treated there, but I felt I could deal with anything, since I had overcome so many obstacles already.

The lecture room where I spoke was well-groomed and elegant. The dark red of the wall-to-wall carpet matched the color of the brick buildings through the white-trimmed windows topped by lunettes. The high ceiling added a sense of space. Comfortable desk chairs were lined in orderly rows. The lectern from which I spoke was on the short side of the rectangular space, daylight entering from the left and opposite walls. I gave a regular, moderate talk that presented my research as somewhat related to biography and carefully avoided theoretical issues and controversies. The participation was high and the atmosphere very cordial, with female graduate students excited about a possible junior professor also female. But at the end of the talk, no challenging questions came my way.

I had meals with several faculty, a female lecturer who had led the basic drama courses and who dressed like a young Southern belle; the coordinator of the recently established women's studies center, who looked more spinsterish and restrained; the token black dean of academic affairs, who looked as if he didn't count and could not care less, his strong, athletic African body bursting at the seams of his three-piece suit and necktie shirt. And of course my chair, a thin, soft-spoken, well-dressed fellow with impeccable Southern manners. He said that no woman had been tenured by the department yet, five junior female faculty having been turned down for unspecified causes. To improve its record, the department had hired a female faculty member in midcareer with tenure from another university. I didn't bat an eyelid, sure that my charm would win them over, and they'd want to redeem themselves with me. The core faculty were of the Agrarian School which celebrated the Old South with its sense of honor and rigid barriers of race, class, and gender. In the Cold War Era, the department had offered New Criticism a home, with its emphasis on the literary text apart from any social or cultural contexts. It now largely lived off its legacy.

As soon as the job offer came, I asked the chair for a one-semester leave without pay. I needed it to go home and get my daughter, Sara, back. "I have a scholarship from the Italian Ministry of Foreign Affairs," I said. Sara was finishing elementary school and would have to change schools anyway. *If I can get myself there quickly enough I can still persuade her,* I thought. The chair explained that I could take a semester off, but it would have to be the second. "Candidates disappear," he said, and it would be best to get to know the department first. I did not explain I had a child abroad, for I was afraid. What about my "past" with a foreigner? Would it come back to haunt me? When my contract letter arrived, it specified that I was free to accept temporary work until the fall, but only "of a respectable sort." The chair, in whose commitment to my appointment I trusted, moved to another school that very summer, never to be heard of again.

VII
Red Marks

As I arrived in Netherville, the languages of my subconscious were still fighting with each other. In the deep summer, the landscape was a rich green deep enough to bring the whole concept of bluegrass to life. Mansions with white-columned porches spread their long, oak-lined entrance drives on the rolling hills of the south pike. It looked like the set of *Gone with the Wind,* women in long, pleated skirts and large straw hats flocking on sunny, green fairgrounds. A lock would brush against a sensuous nape or jaw, its fair gentility protected by a parasol. I had believed this America to be extinct since the Civil War, and wondered what magic brought me into this Hollywood replica. The university was as well groomed and stylish as a plantation home. The flower beds on the quad designed deep greens, pinks, reds, yellows, and purples into lavish ovals. Shapely brick buildings of a dark purple lined the campus's meandering paths, contrasting with the white trim of the windows and tower tops. Rounded shapes promised some baroque indulgence, but the hallways were lined with stern portraits of defunct founders and board members. A moustache turned down, a collar pressing against a jaw, the thick paint of a frock that covered a seemingly wooden flesh announced the austere local elite, and the self-flagellating fundamentalism mixed with agrarian nostalgia which still plagued the university. In the fast-food hangouts around it, whites would not be seen at the table with blacks. No Hispanics or Latinos mediated their face-off. I realized how much I missed the wider diversity of Southern California, how much Latinos had been part of the landscape that made that state feel like home.

I was going to stay for just four months, and made temporary housing arrangements with an acquaintance from UCR, Cynthia's sister, Cheryl. Cynthia had been my first African-American friend in the UCR compound, her daughter, Sharma, was Sara's favorite playmate.

Cheryl was extremely handsome, with an elegance, LA style, that matched her proud deportment. She had a nice condo in a suburban park and was a salesperson for United Airlines who had moved to Netherville from LA on a promotion. She shared stories about getting worn out by the condescendence of her clients, a mixture of misogyny and racism typical of the local mentality.

At my department, colleagues, all male and white, asked me about my housing arrangements and I soon realized that none of them had ever shared their living quarters with a person of color. The janitor of our building was an African American from that area, and I noticed that when he was in the elevator I was the only one to share the ride. I wondered why his eyes would remain lowered, and later learned it was a Southern custom. Lynching was a memory that loomed still large, and a black man would not be found looking a white woman in the eye.

These vestiges of ante-bellum segregation were disturbing enough, buy there was variety among my English colleagues. The liberals, Don Keating and Alfonse Tell, were cordial and debonair. They had interesting marriages, and one would breathe an atmosphere of genteel equality and respect in their families, one blended, the other of the no-kid sort. They were in favor of diversity and moderate political approaches. They welcomed me as a boon to them, but I am not sure they understood me under the political surface. On the other hand, I observed the civility of the hardcore conservatives, who were also married, and who occasionally opened their homes. But their wives seemed to be trained to speak only about lace and silver, and I noticed, from the way they observed my Roman nose, that they seemed to approve of this feat of eugenic distinction. Their stern mien and stiff deportment pointed to their disappointment with the present. They were prepared to accept diversity only if the exotic exemplar was of the most distinguished sort, and I felt clumsy and embarrassed in their homes. Then there were the ultra-confirmed bachelors who usually stayed out of politics, for their alleged queer tendencies were enough of a risk already. I felt a certain affinity for them, for I was by that time tired of straight men. Due to their supposed repression and self-loathing, they were the "other" California's gay culture turned its back to. They were largely unprepared to come out of their closets, and so the AIDS scare caught them unaware. But I found them very tender, and hoped to relax them with my foreignness, an exotic fetish that would enter their fantasy like Judy Garland or Liza Minnelli.

The new elements were a few assistant professors, both male and female, most of whom would quit or be turned down. The one female faculty with tenure from the area had a part-time appointment, and it felt as if she was permanent precisely because she knew her place. She reminded me of Gloria Swanson in *Sunset Boulevard,* a nonliterary version of the faded Southern belle. The midcareer female professor from the Midwest was much more demure and sober. The theorist, freshly hired from the Southwest, was eager to demonstrate his rigor and political correctness. I was not in a good place and so, predictably, I did not connect well. Both my national and my sexual identities were in flux, with my child, the person about whom I was most concerned, on the other side of the ocean. Her life was caught in the quagmire of an undissolved marriage, and my labor certification was still on hold. My inner landscape was undergoing massive transformations and my soul was open to the transpersonal experiences thereof. With a number of colleagues an emotional intimacy was established, and I noticed how the experience of having lived in California, and the shared memories thereof, became the portal to the queer world I longed to explore.

Part of me wondered how I would survive, while I had my mind on getting organized for my leave. In Rome, Sara was starting junior high school, and I was aware of her anxieties about leaving her elementary school and classmates to face new ones. I hoped that my one-semester delay would not cause serious problems in the precarious balance of her life. The apartment my grandfather Gaspare had bought for my mother, Delia, was now empty, for my father had remarried and moved in with Marina. According to the parent-child inheritance laws then in force, it belonged to my brother Andrea and myself. We had arranged for my quasi-ex, Giulio, to live there, as a contribution to his efforts in raising Sara. But I did not want to spend my leave of absence there for I knew it would be unproductive and fraught with risks of reviving a certain construction of Giulio and I as a couple. The scholarship money I would receive was doled out in

Rome on a bimonthly basis, so I could not live too far from the Italian capital, which was, nonetheless, not an ideal location for me for it did not have the right libraries.

I chose Berlin, a small but culturally interesting capital in still-divided Germany, and about twice as cheap as Paris. As a comparatist trained in the old, Eurocentric school, I had learned to admire German music, philosophy, and critical thought, but I could not get past the negative image of German people that came from Nazism. I wanted to know what made my Italian ancestors pick the wrong ally. I already knew three of the four languages that were believed to form the matrix of Western European culture, and wanted to learn the fourth one. The new generation of Germans seemed more humble, and I knew they raised the ecological consciousness of the planet with their hands-off, low energy consumption lifestyles, and the deep-ecology advocacy of their Green Party. German-speaking territory had swallowed both Stephane and José, Francophone as they were. Maybe the children of the nation where Nazism grew had learned a lesson, and on closer look would not resemble their monstrous ancestors. As it turned out, Berlin was both affordable and hospitable. I stayed with the ex-roommate of a Jewish colleague from Netherville, who had also spent time in Germany purging her inner landscape of past hatreds. I also rented a small study, where I did much of the preparation for the theoretical part of my book to come, the revision of my dissertation that—according to the University's regulations—would give me tenure if published on time with an academic press.

Putting this book together turned out to be more difficult than I thought. I knew this enhanced my precariousness, since a whole bunch of people in the department were ready to prey on me. They asked, "Why hire a woman and a foreigner instead of one of our homemade boys, if her performance is not at least stellar?" Indeed, I wondered, *why?* All I wanted to do in my tenure book was point out that there was a problem with monumentalizing the works of modern male playwrights such as Ibsen, Shaw, O'Neill, Miller, and Pirandello, when so many women had been just as good, and just as successful with the public, managing also to bring up issues that were both specific and vital to women's experience, and therefore to humankind. Why were Rachel Crothers, Susan Glaspell, Lillian Hellman, Natalia Ginzburg, and Marguerite Duras not being talked about as much as their male counterparts? Why weren't relationships between women at the center of famous modern plays?

Rather than as a way to get tenure, I saw criticism as a form of justice—literary justice—and wanted to live up to the task. But I was an eclectic in a time of crisis, when it was important to have some bigwig on your side, and when academic presses tended to capitalize on topics that were safe and established, with tiny sensational twists as their spice. I felt that to make my case I had to develop a new theoretical approach, even though I wanted the value of this theory to be shown in the way it applied. This of course, made me a hybrid. "Is she a theorist or a mere critic?" an editor would ask. In my mind, the litmus test was the result of a theory's application. But, as I was wont to discover, this concern was not prominent on most publishers' agendas. I had three strikes against me: I was unknown, my authors were unknown, and my method was unknown too!

True, I had chosen my dissertation topic out of passion rather than political calculation. For example, I did not write about some Renaissance topic, even though my European education gave me great mileage in that area, and still today I am often appalled by the naiveté of some scholars of the early modern era educated on this side of the Atlantic. I also chose not to revise common perceptions of well-known writers in a feminist manner, even though I did know these writers quite well, including Chaucer and Shakespeare. In my mind, that would have been a cop-out to a system that tended to capitalize on what was already powerful, rather than help weaker voices to be heard.

But this was the time of the cultural wars, and, according to the two-party system that characterizes American debate, you had to be either an essentialist or a culturalist. I was both and neither, for my subjects were of the disenfranchised gender, female, and of the dominant race, white. Drama, my genre, had been disenfranchised since New Criticism's heyday. Drama was a political genre, and Cold-War ideology made it unfashionable. Theater was an "impure" art, and a generation of scholars never learned to read plays. But then, the very idea of a genre was too literary according to culturalists—an elitist formalism altogether unnecessary. On top of this, I had my foreign name and accent, which did not inspire publishers much trust. In short, I was on my way to realize that the publication of this book was going to be a long, drawn-out battle, not likely to be over soon enough to appease my enemies. But I had made a commitment to myself and my subject matter, and knew I was going to carry it out.

As my leave ended, I left my Berlin apartment and went back to Rome. It was the summer of 1988, a most heart-breaking and devastating season for me. I felt very proud about myself. Against all odds, I had acquired a professional status in a foreign country, and was ready to share its benefits with those that depended on me, mostly my daughter, Sara. I wasn't sure I would get major accolades and expected nothing like the fireworks that welcomed Stephane when he had returned from France two years earlier. But I thought I deserved some praise. After all, I had done the right thing! Followed the rules, worked hard, made a position for myself, and enfranchised both myself and my child from dependence. Wasn't that something? Well, not so. On my arrival I was immediately assaulted by two major family crises related to my father and daughter respectively. The first one was related to the revelation that for eleven years my father had been in an extramarital relationship with a former flame, Beatrice, one of the many hopefuls Dario had between Delia's death and his second marriage. Beatrice was intense and dramatic, with thick eyeglasses and an ornate style. She had called me many times since Stephane was gone, and I sensed a genuine interest for me. But I believed she and Dario had broken up, and she had turned into an old pal. Now I was learning they had been lovers, and was invited to their new nest. I could explain his wife Marina's long-time hostility to me, probably due to suspicion that I knew of this liaison.

"I felt he had an obligation to tell you," Beatrice said over dinner at a restaurant she had invited me to. "But he wouldn't, so I said I would. I never did before because he threatened to break up with me." I looked at her, incredulous, as she went on, "He loves you too much. You're the only person who can persuade him to divorce his wife."

I thought it was a bit perfunctory to have kept me in the dark for so long and then seek me as an ally. "His two prior wives haven't been especially happy or lucky," I pointed out. "Are you sure it is in your best interest to try?" Beatrice was perplexed by my question and I thought she might have pondered it several times. I felt this whole story was just a way to call attention, for the nth time, to Dario's centrality and the complete marginality of all others within the family orbit.

Andrea and I had decided to sell Delia's house, which was a liability since we didn't live close enough. Giulio had not been able to keep up with the maintenance and I was going for my green card, which meant I might be stuck in the United States for some time. Of course, I would have proposed to change the plans if I knew what was coming. But the second issue confirmed my interpretation of the first one. Having invested a lot of energy in her adjustment to the new school, Sara had made up her mind to stay in it and hence stay with Giulio rather than return to the United States. The whole thing caught me by surprise, and I gradually realized how serious and irreversible it was. I felt somebody with my welfare in mind should have warned me of what was coming. Was I listening? I am not sure. But who would have spoken up? Dario's centrality in the family orbit was in my face one more time.

From the legal viewpoint, I was the parent who had custody, and Sara was too young to make her own decisions. I struggled with her for various weeks as we all stayed in the apartment she and Giulio occupied. The tension mounted. I felt her father should help her evaluate what she was turning down. He, on the other hand, felt he could not abandon her. In his mind, and hers perhaps also, America was this faraway place, strange and ugly, that would swallow Sara up; I was the cruel kidnapper who facilitated that task. I never heard a word of praise for my success, for it was perceived, evidently, as doom and misery for others. It was the very first time I wished I were a man. Surely, my success would have been rewarded in a very different manner. A woman powerful enough to reclaim her child. Parthenogenesis! No phallus necessary! Doom and sadness for the male gender. Since everyone in the family was mired in the crisis, I sought the advice of a professional counselor, and found her through the socialized health-care system. I took Sara there surreptitiously, for both Giulio and Dario thought I would have the counselor manipulate her. She actually advised me not to take Sara away against her will. "You could end up with a suicidal pre-adolescent. Wouldn't that be difficult to manage on your own?" she asked in the stern room of the government building where she practiced.

The country house of my grandmother Teresa was still open, in Fosca, a small town about two hours from Rome. I took Sara there on vacation. No change. Giulio saw his attorney. We ended up in court, and the judge, a woman, empowered Sara to decide which parent she wanted to live with two years ahead of time. I was able to keep both my commitment to my job and the custody, but not the child. In September I made a last attempt to persuade Sara. I went to Bosa, the Sardinian town where she summered with her father's family, and where she had begged me to visit since her father and I had broken up. It did not work, and I remember the azure bay as I rode my taxi to the airport, about one hour away. That driver must have wondered who I was and why I could not stop sobbing. All my life flashed in front of my eyes, and I imagined the way it would have been if I had accepted my destiny of contented Sardinian wife.

I was now definitely a single person. As I returned to Netherville, I was determined to push French and Italian out of my inner landscape. The combat of one subconscious against the others was driving me crazy. Blocking the music of my first native language out of my mind eased the pain of losing my baby. My French lover exited with the second. I was striving for the inversion that would allow American English to envelop these other languages and make its rhythms accessible. It was torture for my inner space. English was never spoken at home, and I had learned it in school, beginning with junior high. But I wanted to use it for my public written expression. It was the colonizer's language, and making it my own would help me reconquer my soul. A colonizer brings women the scent of emancipation and even before 1968 I used to spend time with female schoolmates listening to rock music by the Beatles and Rolling Stones, practicing rock-and-roll and deciphering lyrics, learning jargon and street language.

The Stones were my favorites, for their music was more sensual. "Let's Spend the Night Together" was my favorite song, even though I was still a virgin. For us this music embodied the liberation sought by the *sessantotto,* the movement of 1968.

When I grew up French was still a prominent international language, the only one besides Italian my parents spoke. But English had the makings of an international language, with its worldwide post-colonial circulation. English also had a long tradition of female literary voices whose works were somewhat respected as part of an established canon. One would just have to think of Austen, the Bröntes, Dickinson, and Woolf. Of course, this did not valorize these women as women or feminists, but it gave them a visibility and a role within the context of academic studies the Italian canon had not yet developed.

I had lost my daughter as I pushed my mother tongue out of my inner landscape. As I made progress in my comparative literary studies, English gradually became the language in which I was most well-read, both at the literary and at the philosophical-theoretical level. At that point, I had been teaching basic Italian to native speakers of English for sometime, which had all but mangled my ability to use this language for creative or intellectual expression. I had become used to speaking the Mickey-Mouse Italian that first-year teachers of a foreign language invent to encourage students to believe they can understand, and so avoid falling back on their primary language.

Yet the transition was very complicated. The inversion that brought English to the top of my inner landscape very often felt as a betrayal of my core identity. As a multilingual person, I did have an in-flux identity, but needed a center to hold it together. Italian Americans were still defined as the children of those who came as immigrants with no class privilege or education. They were "the New York Italians" in a way. I didn't quite belong and was too privileged to qualify. But moving to the heartland of America felt like turning my back on my origins, abandoning whatever past I had. And, as I was going to find out, to the Tennessee Agrarians these major differences between Italians were all too subtle.

Between English and Italian stood my French, which had very often interfered with my progress in English, because it somehow tended to impinge on its role as a colonizer's language. When Stephane was in my life, speaking French ruined my chances for a good American-English accent and pronunciation, since its nasal and guttural sounds required the aerobic exercise of specific facial muscles that were useless in any other way. At the same time, French was the witness that I could achieve an imitation almost indistinguishable from the original itself, since I knew for a fact that I could pass for a French person any time I so wished.

My Italian consciousness made me want to go back home; it sucked me back into a pre-Oedipal state as it made me pine for the familiar landscapes, for the sounds of Italian dialects and street talk and folk songs. My French consciousness, on the other hand, made me feel like a perfect fake, who nonetheless would never be part of French society in her own right. My American consciousness was not very strong yet. Its language had a hard time entering the core of my inner landscape, as my English remained abstract, literary. I longed to develop an ear for the regional dialects and inflections, for the idiomatic expressions, the metaphors, the turn of phrases that made American English so rich and fascinating. I was sensitive to their music and longed to play it on my own chords.

The lexical situation was even more topsy-turvy. I was very competent in all the English theoretical, philosophical, and critical terminology. I even had a historical perspective on the language, being able to read and understand both Chaucer and Shakespeare. However, I had no household or kitchen words, and, in English, things as ordinary as a ladle, a saucepan, or even a teapot were nameless for me. It was the same for food textures and flavors like crispy, crunchy, tangy, spicy, and so on, not to mention cooking modes like blend, simmer, poach, steam, or broil.

When my mind worked, my English was grammatically sound and syntactically correct. But this happened only as long as its mode was fear and aggression. The minute I tried another mode, coherence would be lost. This problem reflected my ambiguous relationship with the colonizer at that point in my hybridization process: hatred and resentment still prevailed. We were in the times of George I, of the Bush dynasty, and I was aware of its connections with the CIA. I was reasonably afraid to have a file whose contents would give me up to INS as a red-diaper baby. Would they ask me to repudiate my past? Would they simply reject me with some lame excuse? I knew about the two "Are you now or have you ever been?"s of the process, "homo" and "commie." I had been a member of the Italian Communist Party for a couple of years, before I realized how narrow-minded its sexist leaders were, regardless of their claims. But I also knew that socialist and communist organizations around the globe struggled to be independent of Moscow. In his political career as an independent senator, my father made an emblem of that independence by forcing the PCI, the Italian Communist Party, to let him run in their ticket while he refused to carry their card. The party had done well by pluralizing itself. So much for the first "Are you . . ." I had heard the gloomiest stories about McCarthyism and the red scare, when guilt by association scarred the nation. America had simply not healed and this caused all communisms to appear the same. While in the Eastern bloc voting for a communist party was not a choice, in Italy I knew it was, for there were about a dozen parties. Why did one in three voters choose them? I knew that banning communism for fear it would destabilize democracy was a remedy worse than the problem it claimed to resolve.

As for the other "Are you . . . ," I was unfortunately still completely devoid of confessions to make, since I had never been with a woman or fantasized about it, more than say, noticing how beautiful a certain woman's legs were and wanting to reach out for them with my hand. But I still found the question disturbing. What kind of society was I trying to get into? Was it the sunny, vast, beautiful, spontaneous, and happy America that had seduced my imagination as a girl when I listened to Elvis's "It's Now or Never," the English version of "O' Sole Mio," a famous Neapolitan song? Or was it the conniving, lurking, violent, senseless, and merciless America reflected in the dour mien of Nixon's face? Of course, I didn't know that these two were living together, the doves and the hawks, as Dario used to call them, making, more often than not, quite odd bedfellows. I could only hope that chubby, happy faces spontaneously charming and sensual would come my way, such as those of Marilyn Monroe and JFK, and, eventually, Bill Clinton, the president I would get to vote for my first time at the American polls. It was September 1988, and the university office that was going to process my application for Permanent Residency at Lovelace University declared that I was the best candidate for the job. As I prepared the documents, I could not help feeling proud of myself for having been accepted by this new society on behalf of my professional qualifications. But I was afraid that all my efforts would come to nothing on account of INS-FBI research into the political past of my family. This gave me a sense of nonexistence. I was neither here nor there, and this sense of no place was reflected in my unstable rhetoric. Lucky me, in the world's wider context, the Iron Curtain was falling down and the "Evil Empire" was dissolving. The "Good Empire" was now alone. The system became more lax and the red marks in my consciousness went unnoticed.

VIII
AIDS Scare

The AIDS scare was spreading like wildfire. Now they were telling us that test results could only confirm the absence of infection for the period prior to the past six months. If you tested positive you'd have about five years left. I had been celibate throughout my academic year in Normal, since, to my disappointment, I had discovered that, on a teaching appointment like mine, whomever one met was off-limits for sex. Students, both graduate and undergraduate, were now out-of-bounds. Assistant professors were completely expendable, needles in a haystack of over 200 desperate, overqualified candidates. A student was a precious commodity one was entrusted with. Would one want to be responsible for sending the kid home with the fatal virus? *With these six months of celibacy behind me, I can get a reliable result,* I thought as spring began. I counted my sins. There were a couple of guys I had been with between Giulio and Stephane. One, Nini, was a friend of my brother's. We did it in Andrea's room one day when our apartment in Rome was quite busy with visitors coming and going. I remember that Andrea accidentally caught us in the act, and gracefully closed the door behind himself. Nini had left for Brazil shortly after that, and I remembered his postcard with the sugarloaf Rio mountains, green in the middle of a blue bay. Who had he been with before me? As far as I knew, he certainly could have had some male partners. Then there was of course the Swiss guy with whom I had my fling while still married. He could have been bisexual, and I certainly had no record of his previous partners.

After Stephane I also had had some short flings: the handsome black guy from Trinidad I slept with the night after my last prom ball at Riverside. He told me he was going to get married the next day to a French girl and become a diplomat. He certainly had the looks for it. We had tantric sex, the magic turgidity that keeps, without motion, by the mere force of sacred eroticism. It was the first time for me, almost an accident, as he was also my first black partner. I had my IUD in place, and I'd also use a condom when it was close to expiring. But body fluids were the main lubricants. I thought, *if I came out clean I must have a good star.*

But then, there was the question of my appointment in Netherville. Would it make sense to try to make tenure somewhere if I was going to die? Wouldn't I rather go to a desert island and be inspired to write the lines that would make me immortal, or paint the pictures that the world would admire me for? Wasn't "tenure" a somewhat prosaic project for someone whose lifespan might be as short as that of romantic poets like Keats, Shelley, or Rimbaud? I drove the sixty miles to Champaign for the testing by myself. On the way back, my mind wondered if I would really be able to follow my dreams once my death sentence had been meted out. Wouldn't I, instead, feel depressed and lonely and let myself down to the point that I would carry out that very same sentence? A week later, blessed with a negative verdict, I forgave myself.

But the world we inhabited would not be the same. It would turn into a prison where sex was under siege. The single status I had so ardently earned was going to be the way I would serve my time. My best relationships had developed out of spontaneous sexual expression, starting as one-night stands that evolved if the time and place were right. To me, the guarded courtship that characterized the love life of women like my mother was totally foreign. I knew Delia had intentionally raised me to be wired this way. Courtship was a thing of the past, with pursued and pursuer clearly defined, with moderate erotic contacts gradually permitted as the "serious intentions" solidified, and with the bride as a pristine package to be unwrapped on the wedding night. I knew my body enough to be aware of its erotic impulses, and when the chemistry was right, I just went ahead and acted on them. I was a good lover for I had gotten good training and was generous enough to pass it around. I considered lovemaking the most sophisticated and healthy of all arts. Now people were scrambling to get fixed up with a suitable partner, even if he or she was the lousiest lover they ever had, and then proceeded to fence themselves out in their safe monogamy garden. Stephane, I felt, was doing the same, despite his lapse when we made love that summer of 1988. I wasn't cut for the game, and fared on the wayside which was a penance, and I still wonder if the lessons were worth learning. .

The second time I got tested was in Netherville, for immigration the next fall. The AIDS test was included in the mandatory checkup, and the nurse said its results would not affect my application. This time I had not much to worry about, but wondered, had I turned out "infected," would the system still have approved of my green card? I was not aware of false positives and cross reactions, which were documented later, by AIDS dissenters. My blood was clean enough, but, had I been dealt a false positive, would I have been strong enough to offset its lethal charge? My thoughts went to my late mother and other victims of medical hexing unable to exorcize their curse.

As I looked around myself, I realized that in the late 1980s, at the peak of the AIDS scare, three cultures shared a living space in the city of Netherville. In this predominantly white urban area one could find a social elite in the style of the Old South, an active population gravitating around the main production centers of the pop music industry, and an educational community intent in mediating their somewhat difficult relationship. The rather stable upper-middle class was fundamentalist and mostly made of nuclear families. The music industry population, with a higher share of transient elements, was regarded by conservatives as potential clientele for the local prostitution industry. The university that hired me was a private institution mainly devoted to educating the children of the affluent regional elite. At this time, however, it was also in the process of establishing a national reputation by diversifying junior faculty and attracting "stars" with its endowed chairs. Although somewhat besmirched by its racist Agrarian past and by its conservative New Critics legacy, the English department had a good reputation and several good professors. I was just a beginner, but, as a non-Anglophile foreigner, I would certainly tip the balance in favor of the diversification project. In addition, I would bring the institution some diversification funds from the Federal Government, which would stay with the institution whether they kept me or not.

Inevitably, the university's modernization project clashed with the AIDS scare. The fear of infection had crossed the boundaries of the gay male community and was spreading all over the place. God-fearing souls saw this health crisis as deserved retribution for the lavish fruition of sexual pleasure brought about by the liberalism of the previous decade. To be spared was all they wished for themselves and their relatives. For many liberals of all sexual orientations, the fear of getting infected turned into a desire to learn and disseminate knowledge about safer sex, by which it could assuage the incipient panic. But within the institutions of law and order, this fear generated an unprecedented belligerence against all kinds of unsanctified, nonlegitimate sex. In several medium-size cities of the United States, the police, encouraged by public outrage, ran campaigns designed to eradicate sexual activities involving an exchange of money and those performed in public spaces.

Some newly acquired faculty members came from large metropolitan areas where the police did not have time for minor offenses, and where, throughout the 1960s, the 1970s, and most of the 1980s, educational and social communities had been open spaces for sexual play—both straight and gay. But now, any kind of on-campus sexual expression was subject to being constructed as either sexual harassment or rape, and the police were coming down on all kinds of casual or semicasual sex. The newcomers must have felt so lonely and bereft of congenial spaces for sexual play, that some of them resorted to the local prostitution industry. As a teaching assistant, I had fallen in love with my own student in a one-night stand that developed into a six-year relationship. How could I not sympathize with them?

The stings were designed to entrap members of a disenfranchised minority, with undercover agents placed at strategic points in the cityscape. In Tennessee, the old sodomy laws were still in place and this made accosting a same-gender prostitute a felony. In that AIDS-scare climate, it was easy to pass these cleansing operations as legitimate and necessary. Perceived as the victim of, and cause for, the spread of AIDS, the gay male population was classified as a special-target risk group. In many cases, the decoy for the sting was a young man, just barely under age. The voices of his would-be clients were taped, and these persons were then identified and arrested, with attached listing of their names in the local papers. Even though at least one of my colleagues was a victim of this kind of entrapment, I found out about them one year later, when I had already sold my property in Rome, bought a house in Netherville, and lost my child.

While still in the job market, I had already experienced some serious AIDS-scare frustration. With sexuality being my only access to the sacred, and my French partner gone, I felt withdrawal from lack of opportunities to get the kind of casual or semicasual sex I had sometimes enjoyed. The victims had all my sympathies since I felt they were only doing what comes naturally and seemed logical now that university regulations tended to criminalize all casual sex. Yet the situation scared me because the topic was kept under wraps and only alluded to in surreptitious ways. I believed sodomy to refer exclusively to anal pleasure, and was not aware of its being legislated. I also took for granted that no legal restrictions would apply to the positions in which consenting and grown sexual players chose to enjoy their erotic pleasures. Now, I was getting a crash course in sodomy law and criminal conversation while I was already in a situation where even proffering an interest in sex could land one in jail. All of a sudden my liberalism in erotic expression appeared criminal even to myself. My sexual impulses froze, and I embarked on a dire two-year celibacy spell.

Even as I had more white hair than is common in one's thirties, I wanted to assuage any fears my employers might have about "redheads." During my last year in town I had met a foreign student from Eritrea. He spoke Italian and was black. He was in economics, a department far enough from mine to make him eligible for sex of the amorous but noncommittal sort. Yet my fears ran so deep I felt my amorous life was over, and I turned him down many times for sex. It took all of his patience to break my celibacy spell. There was ethnic strife in East Africa but no news came because the media was focused on the Gulf War. One day he came home overjoyed. He had finally got word that his relatives were safe. I had died my hair red again for I was getting ready to move to California. When we finally did it, I cried for joy.

When I learned about the entrapments, I was appalled by the police methods not only because they violated the civil rights of the indicted persons, but also because, as an educator, I felt the use the police made of the minors they employed was highly questionable. Weren't these young decoys potential members of an ideal, non-exclusionary, learning community in their own right as well? Sure, their dads could not afford the tuition fees our university charged, but I felt they deserved to learn what life is all about in a more honest and dignified way.

The university's law school had a very good reputation and it could have expressed its outrage against the police behavior. But, instead of taking an active role in the making of public policy, the institution swept the garbage under the rug, and bought the silence of its employees with the threat of associating them with the unpleasant notoriety of the indicted persons. This was the first example of a major erosion of human dignity and respect in the social fabric and workplace that affected me directly since I moved to the New World. It was the end of a dream, and the awakening was a shock for which I could not have been remotely prepared. It was as if the backdrop of the New World stage had suddenly fallen, to expose the corruption and miserliness in which persons in power and practitioners of political correctness engaged.

IX
The Making of Knowledge

These were my early years as an assistant professor, and I believed in the educational system because it had rewarded me even as I gradually learned to play its game. As a befitting daughter to a political reformer and an experimental pedagogue, I felt a good educational system functions like a filter between social structures and new generations. Even though we are not all born equal, a fair and accessible educational system can enable those with merit to get ahead, and so make sure that the cosmos falls in good hands. I saw crime, the mafia, and other social problems as the result of an educational system's failure to propel exuberant creative energy into socially productive directions. *Al Capone was not an idiot,* I used to think to myself, *and I'm sure his creative intelligence could have been used in much better ways!* As a graduate student, I had been trained to despise teaching and to be research obsessed, even though part of me never really saw it that way. In my imagination, the classroom was a shared research laboratory, and every act of learning was an act of discovery, a self-teaching process in which the learning community engaged. I saw my research as the simple act of transcribing the experience of facilitating this process, and so I thought of the two processes as interdependent and complementary. These ideals had been cultivated in Riverside, which had initially functioned for me as a quasi utopian space.

But the system did not see things that way. My first years out of graduate school were the years of the cultural wars, when the system was coming to terms with the end of modernity, the fact that there was going to be no endless progress toward a better tomorrow. The aftermath of modernity can be interpreted in various ways. The Italian philosophers of the *pensiero debole* believe that we need to develop a thought style that reflects a position of weakness rather than strength. At the end of modernity, they say, giving up traditional reason and logic is both convenient and necessary. "Strong" thought proceeds from the mind, with sight as its preferred mode of knowledge. It has prevailed throughout modernity, even as it was invented much earlier. "I came, I saw, I conquered," said Julius Caesar, the first Roman emperor. "I came," so my eyes saw and my mind mapped out the situation. The war began, and it ended with the conquest of the enemy. This thought is based on what moderns call "reason." The irony is that, in the postmodern age, *this* reason is not reasonable at all. We've conquered the planet over and over; there's nothing left. And if we don't stop depleting the earth's resources, Gaia, as ecofriendly scientists like to call the sum of the atmosphere and biosphere, will conquer us by turning back into a rock or at least a place inhabited only by bacteria and other unicellular organisms. The end of modernity thus forces a change in epistemological perspectives. Now, Western thought looks neither superior nor universal. Just one among many. While in the past it might have worked, at least for some, from now on it won't work at all.

For "strong" thought, acquiring knowledge is like waging a war. Just like my Roman ancestors, the scholar who wants to know violently invades, plunders away, and finally subdues the "field" or territory assigned to himself or herself. This done, the knower fences the field off, configures it in a more or less organized way, and allows in only those who are willing to cultivate it for him or her. The scholar fends off any foreign invaders, namely any attempts to change the configuration of the territory.

This system, of course, does not facilitate collaboration, and is, therefore, an obstacle to any practical or providential utility or progress, except, of course, in the sense of accruing power to those in control. The ethics of this process have always been questionable. But at the end of modernity, our species has the power to destroy, not only all possible human adversaries, but also a portion of the earth's mantle teeming with life large enough to render our very existence impossible. Consuming more energy in adversarial endeavors only serves to come closer to the point of no return. The conquest of new knowledge is hopelessly unsustainable, and participating in it is dangerous and senseless. But fortunately, there are alternative epistemological modes that emphasize knowledge by touch and connectedness, collaboration among those involved, and respect, reverence, and contemplation for those or that which we hope to know.

Most of us who entered the edifice of knowledge in the late 1980s wanted to remodel the building in some way. Some negotiated new territory with the intent of raising parallel or perhaps opposed temples. For example, we chose to study bodies of writing that had so far been ignored, in the hope that these very same bodies would point the way to reforming the epistemology that had caused the exclusion in the first place. These bodies were the writings of humans disenfranchised by gender, race, sexuality, age, culture, nationality, ability, and a host of other factors that positioned them in a situation from which new horizons could be discerned. In my case, the body of virtually unknown works were the plays by women of the modern era, and by examining them I discovered what axiomatic concept had rendered them invisible in the first place, what preconceived notion of drama had made them forgettable. Instead of a phallic hero engaged in an action that was mimetic of a man's orgasm, that has its very same rhythm and shape, their dramatic structure was based on a dual protagonist made of two female characters interconnected like labia. This figure of two-in-one presented a new mimetic mode which was labial like one of the ways in which women experience pleasure, and opened a whole new range of epistemological modes apt to constructing the relationship between experience and the intelligible in ways that empowered the weak subjects it represented. The weakness of these subjects was the source of their strength for they knew how to live with less of those shared resources others were consuming at a dangerously fast pace. Negotiating new territory was risky, but there was merit in the shared effort of trying to get out of modernity in a safer way.

Others wished to inhabit the main building, and simply redecorate it. They were content with studying the monuments of modernity again, such as Shakespeare, Pirandello, and Henry James. They delighted in looking at them from a slightly different angle. For example, they examined the way sexual desire was displayed in their works, hoping to point to some of the limitations of the prevalent epistemological mode that would perhaps correct it or improve it in some way. I don't think this position was very brave. As explorers, we were out to not only bring back into the realm of the knowable what had been excluded by a limited epistemology, but also to reconfigure the disciplines to which this knowledge was apportioned, as a way to raise serious questions about the nature of knowledge and the process by which it is created. But the redecorators thought of us explorers as "positivist," and therefore unable to really challenge the established methods. To those of us who charted new moldable spaces, the leaders in the remodeling program were acting as patriarchy's precious children, who entered the master's house to establish their claim to a share of the cultural capital at hand. Of course, each side accused the other of being essentialist and politically incorrect, while the conservative impulse to privatize education fed on the public's sense of confusion with respect to the debate.

In my view, a new theory had no value as long as its pragmatic necessity hadn't been demonstrated. Therefore, negotiating new territory meant applying a hypothesis to a previously unanalyzed body of work, and find out what new theory developed thereof. It was the process of finding out which theory was comfortable and capable of creating a wholesome learning space that demonstrated its worth. For example, Lacan's theory that there is no pre-Oedipal, no prediscursive dimension of existence made me very uncomfortable. I thought of beings that have no discourse, or whose discourse is not intelligible to humans, such as dolphins, ants, dogs, stones, or waves. Who are we to say that we are better than they are? Are we really sure that their prediscursive life is nonexistent or nonimportant? On the other hand, the French feminist philosopher Luce Irigaray proposes an epistemology that privileged the sense of touch as a mode of knowledge. Her attention to the kind of nearness between distinct beings that almost erases the distinction between them, her representation of the self as two-in-one rather than just one, felt very cozy. If successful, the application of these hypotheses would open new possibilities and dimensions, which, in my view, were necessary to heal from modernity and its diseases, from its blindness to the limitations and dangers of its prevalent epistemological mode. And in my appointment, I intended to practice them and profess them.

The kind of knowledge that interests me and interested me then is gnoseologic in the sense that it comes as much from observation of the external world as from self-knowledge, and is, therefore, initiatory, creative, and transpersonal. I was searching for a part of myself I did not know, both in discursive and erotic expression. And so when I arrived at the university I was looking for a mentor, an interlocutor who would also function as a portal to the worlds I did not know. UCR was well-known for its progressive pedagogy and I had had very good professors, but something was still missing. I wanted to nurture my creative impulses as much as my scholarly ones, and for some reason I thought that to become a writer you had to meet a man who was a writer, and one whose writing you admired, and hope that he would take an interest in yours. This would mean support during the struggle for getting your first work together, and access to the publishing world, which I believed to be governed by the laws of male complicity and misogynist friendship. And indeed, as far as I knew, it was. Who had helped the female writers the public at large was aware of, if not their male mentors? Dacia Maraini and Alberto Moravia, Lillian Hellman and Dashiell Hammett, Franca Rame and Dario Fo, Simone de Beauvoir and Jean-Paul Sartre, Anaïs Nin and Henry Miller, and so on and so forth. I did believe that these women had merits of their own, and knew that they had eventually broken away from the male tutelage that helped them get going. Yet I was simply convinced that finding that kind of tutelage was necessary.

And so I was looking for a mentor, who, at least in my imagination, was two things in one. He was the male energy behind my struggle to complete my first book, and the possessor of the key to the publishing world that would pry open that door for me. My professors had been generous with their attention, yet for some reason I was not done yet. As my different cultural legacies fought with one another for possession of my soul, I was searching for my own voice in the English language. I had read the books of my well-published professors, but none struck me as somebody whose talent was strong enough to have made a living out of his pen. While I certainly did not expect critics to write pulp novels, I was looking for a strong individual voice—a cultural analyst and narrator whose books I could not put down, for they would read better than the fictional works therein discussed. As my grandmother used to say, he or she who cannot do the work cannot supervise it either *(chi non lo sa fare non lo sa comandare),* which was a way for Fosca's peasants to get back at the inept landowners they sometimes served. Based on Teresa's wisdom, I was prepared to unconditionally admire a scholar only if he or she had a narrative vein of his or her own, for I felt only this would make that person a fair, compassionate commentator of other people's work.

The feminist consciousness I had developed in Italy in the 1970s—during the divorce and abortion campaigns—led me into my journey for a California graduate education, and the research plan on female writers I developed there. I was proud to be a feminist. And I admired many American feminist scholars, theorists, and activists who would have made terrific mentors had I been lucky enough to know them. But there were good reasons why in my imagination this mentor was a male. As a foreign woman of some sex appeal and known to be heterosexual, I had not been able to develop network of female friends. On the straight side, most white American women I came in contact with saw me as a rival and a disloyal person. My Italian manners appeared seductive to them, and their mixture of envy and contempt for the presumed power these manners gave me was an obstacle to our relatedness. On the gay side, of course, I might have looked interesting to some lesbians, but they regarded my cultural background as too homophobic to consider the project of undertaking my initiation to their ways. I did not yet know any Italian-American women, nor any women from Italy who had recently moved to the United States. At UCR, my female friends and interlocutors had been the Francophone émigré Geraldine; the African-American math student, Cynthia, mother of Sara's playmate; and Karen, a Jewish-American independent scholar married to my professor B. J. These women were barely making it themselves, and it was hard for me to see them in a mentorial role. Furthermore, in my department all professors with power and ascendancy over graduate programs were male, with the only woman—whose advice I sought when I met Stephane—relegated to undergraduate education. No wonder I was hooked on male energy as far as mentoring styles were concerned!

I had this obscure notion that good writers had a special way to connect their physical person to the voice that came off from the page, whether their specialty was fiction, biography, drama, philosophy, poetry or all of the above. I imagined that if I could only meet one such person and come to know him intimately and directly, for some reason miraculously that connection would happen for me also. While I knew I could write English and teach it correctly, I was also aware that I was too dependent on its grammatical rules to bend it to my expressive needs, to accommodate the kind of vernacular expression that makes a piece ring true. This limitation was like a straitjacket. I could function simply as an instrument for the transmission of knowledge, I could not twist or bend it my own way. My imagined mentor would give me permission for my transgressions, so I would come into my own.

I found what I wanted even though I sometimes wished I had not because the challenge was often too strong. Gnosis is a mode of knowledge based on love, and it sometimes demands unconditional love. It is often practiced in response to the dysfunctional medicalization of love produced in mainstream psychotherapy discourse. I received the knowledge I wanted and found the self-knowledge I was looking for, even as I learned to surrender to this practice in the process.

My appointment at Lovelace was my first experience in private education. In elementary school, my mother, Delia, had me driven to the other side of town in order to attend the only public Montessorian school in Rome. And I loved the space of free inquiry, rapt attention, and intense analysis the Montessori classroom offered; the expansive joy of learning; teachers who rarely taught and quietly allowed the learning process to unfold; students who chose their own assignments and were expected to help others learn; the ultimate punishment being to be kept from learning. I credit that early romance with learning and teaching as what has sustained me throughout my life in education, and its miseries. Besides, at least in my time, private schools in Italy were almost invariably Catholic, and my parents thought a child should not even read the Bible lest she or he be exposed to the dogma of the "one true church." But there was more; my mother felt that teachers are accountable not only to their students and principals, but also to the society that their students will contribute to as adults, often in capacities of power to which their degrees entitle them. The only way to ensure that double accountability was a public entity, a *res publica,* as it was called in the Roman republic era, that mediated the relationship between those subject to being educated and the society their learning would enable them to serve. This *res publica,* this public entity was an evenly funded, largely centralized, and free of charge system of public education. Delia was wont to make comparisons with the Romans, and she used to tell me of the slaves patricians enfranchised based on their learning, so that they could be assigned to the tutoring of their children. They were often from Greece, which the Romans considered their cultural matrix. These tutors, she claimed, never taught what was tough or controversial, for they'd be sent right back to the slave quarters. The result was obtuseness and ignorance of those in control, a major reason why the Roman Empire gave way. Of course, there was nothing wrong with that collapse per se, but a more competent ruling class would have secured a softer landing. At Lovelace University, I felt I would be in the uncomfortable position of those Greek tutors in the Roman patrician families. Would I help the crumbling empire hold together, or would I watch while it fell on its face?

I set out to teach my assigned classes, a freshmen course of introduction to drama and expository writing, and three upper-division courses in European, American, and British drama, respectively. Of course, I had no sense of how much students hated freshman writing, since I had always taught language classes, which were usually fun. Nor could I identify with the authoritarian ways in which they knew how to learn. I had learned to write in Italy, where elegance and style were considered the mirror of a position's inner value. And I knew nothing about learning styles in which responsibility was not shared. At Lovelace, I felt miserable in class and was not satisfied with my performance. But the pain of the experience was nothing compared to the devastating way in which the department dealt with it.

For one thing, when the time of my second-year review came, no one wanted to be on the committee to evaluate me. They had lured me away from my child, country, and lover, gotten me back to the United States, and declared I was the best possible candidate so my green card application could be processed. Now it was time to get my contract renewed and they didn't even care. Perhaps my colleagues did feel that something didn't click in my life, that I was not happy. But then, wouldn't that be a reason to lend a hand? I began to appreciate Catholicism, for in a Catholic culture I would not have been abandoned that way.

Then there were the student evaluations. I will not forget the humiliation of reading the xenophobic and misogynistic remarks that were not edited for teaching content, and contained, still in student handwriting, depressing and insulting comments. A student asked, "Why does Lovelace have to go all the way to Italy to find teachers of English?" Another remarked, "Dr. Cosentini is a brilliant woman with a less than brilliant ability to teach." Recognizing a student's handwriting was part of the frustration, for I could be attacked, but could hold no one responsible. In general, my evaluations were about two points below what I had always gotten in Italian, which was about half a point below the top.

I didn't realize what a test it was for these privileged students from a provincial Southern town to have me teach them the language they believed to be theirs by birthright. My diction was clear, but I often used a low tone of voice out of reverence for the subject matter and to facilitate their autonomous thinking processes. To defuse my authority and empower them, I often had students sit in a circle rather than the more conventional rows. Of course, my mild accent denoted me as a foreigner, which to them meant untrustworthy. How would they respect me as a source of authority? For me, the classroom performance was a test of how genuine the institution's commitment to me really was, and to the diversification project I represented. When I read those comments, I was floored with grief and sadness, and knew not what to say. I thought the chair or dean would call me in their office to offer their apologies and find a way to cheer me up. If not, I thought, "What's the point of having me here?" After all, Netherville was a small place, even for the scions of the upper crust. Were their limitations going to determine who could teach at the university that was supposed to broaden the horizon of their imagination? By exposing them to a host of models one could hope to pierce through the deep-seated prejudices they absorbed in their native environments, and prepare them for higher responsibilities. But no. As I discovered, the dean was worried that, as a result of having hired me, some of these precious kids would spend their trust funds in some other institution.

The chair asked me to form my own committee, since everybody he knew was reviewing somebody else. I was left to my own devices. All the drafts I was editing were exposed to the entire department as proof of my incompetence. All of a sudden, my classes were full of visitors testing my teaching skills. No advice, no comfort came about the harsh treatment from the students. The committee presented my case to the department in a negative way. They found all possible reasons to blame me. A trilingual journal from Italy that published in Italian, English, and French had accepted an English article of mine. The galleys showed hyphenating errors neither I nor the typesetter had caught. Surely, that was wrong, but why not look at this journal's effort to accommodate me? How many American typesetters can even set a sentence of Italian without major mistakes? The committee could have considered that. But no. After only three semesters of unsupervised work, I was found "deficient" in both teaching and research. There were only two votes in my favor. My contract was terminated and I had a year's time to find myself another job. I filed a grievance and kept the process going for another semester. The committee was asked to evaluate its own procedure, which it did, confirming its prior decisions.

I had another year in the initial contract to figure out what went wrong. Much as I had wanted to teach English, I was now beginning to realize that to these students, as well as to other American undergraduates, English was not the language of rebellion against the establishment Italian students like me learned in the 1960s, to the tunes of our favorite rock songs. To them, it was like a prison. In their monolingual education it was the only language in which a vast majority of them could actually experience life. And, with expository writing being the type of written expression the educational system primarily valued, they associated writing with a set of regulatory codes permeated with ideology. As I learned in teaching the freshman classes, the ideology I had to instill was problematic for me. Writing was arguing like an attorney, defending your client. This rhetorical strategy based on litigation had war as its main avenue; conquest its goal. It only stiffened the soul and expended valuable creative energies into an adversarial struggle. My colleagues had suggested that I read their rhetoric's little bible, a manual of style written by two typically waspish guys by the last names of Strunk and White. I can't forget their maxim: "no useless words!"

White had been Strunk's student, and he had turned out to be an exact copy of the master, with both men forming the perfect example of an Irigarayan hom(m)osexual couple, a pair in which all genders and sexualities have been perfectly homogenized to the dominant one; a complicity that put any diversity out of sight. Of course, *No useless words,* I thought, *but where does one draw the line?*

When I was a child, Western movies were a popular genre, if cheap—not my favorite. Their heroes, usually tough redneck cowboy types, easily replaced all words with guns. They were emblems of Reagan's America, and its thirst for conquest in a regime of unmitigated capitalism. As I remembered myself laughing at this ridiculous argument, I knew which words must have seemed useless to Strunk and White. The ideology I had failed to teach my classes was that time is money, and there must be pleasure neither in reading nor in writing. I wondered why I had never heard of this manual before. But I was grateful to my professors at Riverside for sparing me, and making me feel more at home by teaching Barthes's *The Pleasure of the Text.* What about seduction, gradual unveiling, a style of criticism that has a story, passion, flair—European style? No! I had to direct students to get right down to their thesis. I was clearly at odds with myself and the way I experience writing, and wondered, *Who would want to read an entire paper if the whole content is given away in the first paragraph?*

In the literature courses, I was up against the legacy of New Criticism, which exonerated students from learning much about the context of literature, its history and politics. This legacy loomed large in that glory of the Old South, that hub of the not-quite defunct Agrarians. This explained why the drama courses of the English department to which I had been assigned had not been taught for a while. I had also been up against a prevalent teaching mode based on authority, according to which teachers did all the teaching, and students did all the learning there is to do in a class. Roles were etched in stone, never exchanged or reversed. Knowledge was just passed from a higher to a lower station, never generated from peer collaboration or self-guidance. I had conducted these courses as seminars, in which students were responsible for part of class time, giving reports on both group and individual assignments. In their evaluations, several students observed that I wasn't earning my money, for they were doing my job!

Indeed, my mother might have been right, and we professors of the good empire were just cultured slaves who had earned our freedom so as to be more dignified as tutors of an elite that had power no matter how ignorant it was.

The English department was in the midst of the cultural wars that swept across the nation. Specialties defined in traditional ways were considered "essentialist," including literary periods or movements like Romanticism and Victorianism, centuries like the eighteenth century, and authors like Shakespeare. The culturalists complained that their disciplinary approach was essentialist, in the sense that it implied a predetermined notion of their study area, which per se prevented more open-ended speculations. Other disciplines defined as area studies, such as Gender, Neocolonial, or Early Modern Studies, were considered to have a social constructionist philosophical base, precisely because they did not imply such predefined notions. Modern drama, my specialty, was defined by period, of course, and by genre, which is a literary category. So it fell into the essentialist camp in some ways, even though, of course, I was not an advocate of conservative doctrines, and I had chosen it precisely because, in its relatedness to the practice of theater, drama is less purely literary than other genres like the novel or poetry. But, given the situation, the specialty defined me, and, ironically, on the part of social constructionists, there was no attempt to look beyond predetermined ideological bases upon which appointments were made.

These rather basic philosophical debates had been taking place as a recessive economy and technological expansions in cyberspace chipped away at the last vestiges of the progress made by the labor movement that developed in response to the industrial revolution. These were based on the principle that workers are not slaves but dignified human beings with a right to think for themselves and be protected from injustice. They included a sense of respect for personal dignity, for intellectual and spiritual independence, and for the wisdom that comes with experience and age. The transient labor force that resulted from this effort was entirely controllable and expendable, as it was prey to the global market's fluctuations. In this new era of postmodern nomadism, the fear of being reduced to a transient state made it seem most noble of those consumed in walking the politically correct tightrope to engage in a modest remodeling of the edifice of culture. Their sense of heroism prevailed, even as the expenses of their modest progress were paid by those intent in exploring new areas and modes of knowledge altogether. So the women whose intellect grew in the aura of new feminism now banked on capital's master texts, Shakespeare's and James's, and bought an entrance ticket to the patriarchal structure by looking at the canon from a slightly different angle. They sold their sisters down the river by riding bigger horses that ran faster and took them more quickly to the end of the race. They did nothing new of their own; they secretly despised female writers and indirectly contributed to their obfuscation. They believed that you can learn about women in the Renaissance by just looking at what Shakespeare wrote about them, ignoring what women in Shakespeare's time, such as Mary Roth, Laura Cereta, Louise Labé, Veronica Franco, and many others had done to leave a testimony of their experience behind themselves.

Of course, the redecorators did not challenge the existing disciplinary configuration for it would threaten the stability of their career path, and their ability to access grant money and other resources. But the manner in which disciplines are configured on the map of knowledge that each age considers right is both a reflection and a result of prevalent epistemological styles. The current map that redecorators left unchallenged was precisely the one that mirrored Western epistemology that constructs knowledge as a form of conquest. Political correctness was thus turned on its head, for those who claimed authority on the basis of their ability to challenge the status quo ended up accepting it instead.

I held English departments in high esteem, for I had been an English major as an undergraduate in the Italian university system. As a comparatist in my graduate education I had not become aware of how most English professors in the United States were monolingual and encouraged to stay that way, with translation being so poorly rewarded as academic work. My languages lived with me as they continued to inhabit my inner landscape in their usual promiscuous ways. I suppose my colleagues felt both estranged from and threatened by my interlinguistic discourse production process. My interaction with them was fraught with contradictions, yet it did empower me to use English as my language of public expression. As for the South, as a culture and bioregion, I left with the curiosity to know more and with the fear of being stigmatized as diverse.

At the end of my last semester at the university, I moved to Southern California. I had decided I was going to spend the next chapter of my life in a less xenophobic, more erotically empowering place. I dreamed of oceans, reminding myself that the French word for ocean also means mother, *la mèr/e,* and obscurely feeling that the secret of my voice was in finding my connection to that body of water again. I drove across the country to the San Diego area. Strong with the lessons of LA's pollution blowing over to Riverside, I was determined to live with no carbon dioxide blown on my face. Once there, I rented an oceanview duplex in Cardiff, a beach town north of La Jolla. Nearby Encinitas was a major holistic center. I drove to its beach and lay down on the shore pebbles. The waves whooshed through them, and I listened to Gaia, the earth, breathe under my belly.

X
Coming to Bisexuality

As I drove on Interstate 40, in that summer of 1991, I felt the energy of the dream that made me move back to the West flow into my brain again. The last months in Netherville had been an agony of decision making. What would the next chapter be? What direction would my life take? Then the interview for my green card came, and I knew I had a choice. I did not consult Dario, Andrea, Beatrice, or Sara back home, for I knew they would urge that I return to Italy.

The Pacific represented a total freedom of the imagination, the last shore where the West could still afford to dream itself beautiful and fair, the grassroots, hippie America whose wonder had captured my mind as a teenager, and from which ivory-tower prisons supposedly kept one away. San Diego was a border city, its biculturalism self-evident in the way Mexican and WASP cultures cohabitated. Its hills and meandering bay had attracted San Francisco Bay Area radicals from the hippie days. And the military base gave its basic conservatism a queer taste.

In the fall, I volunteered at what was then called the Gay and Lesbian Center in downtown San Diego. I thought I'd be able to find out more about AIDS. I was assigned to a safer-sex education unit. Robin, the organizer, was a critical-care nurse who lived in North County like me. I went to her place in denims and a white blouse, a fabric rose in my cleavage, no bra. She got me involved in preparing safer-sex kits for teach-ins at the Metropolitan Community Church and other sex-positive organizations. She explained all about the exchange of fluids and the risk of infection and showed me how to turn a condom into a dental dam. Then we decided to try it.

Robin dreamed of a highly sanitized world in which women were completely self-sufficient, and men were kept at bay. She had a rather medicalized idea of parenting, and told me about her dream of performing artificial insemination on her partner some day. She was very sweet and chubby, preferring oral sex, and must not have found me very adept, since I was a bit hesitant, and not quite content with the 100 percent protection she demanded. She allowed me to penetrate her with my latex-gloved fingers and it felt completely different from anything I'd tried before. A woman, with her cavity, with her hole, just like me. The hole was in front of me; it wasn't me. And the hole was not a hole, it was an organ with its vibrant flesh, with its turgidity and sensations. Finally, I had broken the sound wall, I was on the other side of experience, I knew who I was for I knew one who was like me.

In June 1992, Sara and her friend Laura came to visit for about two months. It was extremely stressful, for they were teenagers and wanted to go out every night. They were not interested in anything but discos and nightclubs. For underage people those were open only from 2 a.m. on, and so I had to drive them downtown and then pick them up at the wee hours of the morning. Robin invited the three of us to prepare more kits, and I welcomed the opportunity to give Laura and Sara some safer-sex education too. They listened and cooperated.

It was time for the Gay Pride Festival, and with Robin we manned the booth on lesbian safer sex. It was a great opportunity to get to know the gay, lesbian, bisexual, and transgender community in its diversity, a community in transformation whose new and expanded acronym, GLBT, was going to express exactly that. There was music at night and Renée and I sat watching from the rows. I thought, *This is more like falling in than coming out. If I become a lesbian, what do I make of my past? I've had so much fun with men in bed. Could I repudiate that? Pretend it never happened? I'll lose part of myself and sooner or later I'll feel sorry about it.* Sara and Laura were having fun dancing with each other. I thought they figured out what was happening and were having a try at it on their own. Eventually they went back home, and I realized I still grieved for not having Sara more in my life. Difficult as it was, I was deluded to think that if she had been under my supervision all the time, her teenage rage, her growing-up pains would not have been so hard to endure.

At the Pride festival I walked up to a booth that said bisexuality. A Frenchman said "hallo," and I recognized the accent. So I told him *"Je parle Français,"* and we started to talk. He told me all about his organization, the Bi Forum, and invited me to the next monthly meeting. I went and immediately felt I had found a new family. It was like coming home in a very deep and unmistakable way. Despite the support-group atmosphere, people seemed to really know and like each other, like a large family or a tribe. They encouraged newcomers to speak out and many brought up their issues. A man in a gay relationship was seeing a woman on the side, and his boyfriend found out. A woman was married and found out her husband was seeing guys. One woman in a committed relationship with another woman, fell for a guy. A man in a threesome with a woman and a man had been dumped by both partners. How do you deal with these situations? What do you recommend? What role models do you have? How do you make these persons feel who they are is all right? What measures of safety and responsibility do you recommend?

The veterans in the group were really great at sharing their experiences. They all had "been there done that," got out of it all right, and lived to tell the tale. Now they knew what to do about it. It was phenomenal. Finally I wasn't alone and there was nothing wrong with me and what happened to me all my life was all right! The group discussed issues like nonmonogamy and disclosure of one's sexual orientation to partners. Another emphasis was setting boundaries of safety that would make sexual partners feel comfortable. For example, one would have a primary partner, with whom fluids were exchanged, and secondary partners with whom latex barriers were used. Honesty and negotiation were always recommended, including those about emotional and physical safety. I did bring up my issues with Stephane, including the fact that I had desired his girlfriends and felt betrayed that they liked him, not me. At the end of the meeting the monthly social was announced, and one could pick up an invitation. Robin came to one meeting, but declared she didn't like the group and wouldn't come back. She gave me an ultimatum, either them or me. I chose them.

At a lesbian social I learned about the Equal Employment Opportunity Commission from a friend of Robin's who was an attorney. I knew that in the United States the judicial system was easier to activate than in Italy, where litigation was infrequent because of the excessive slowness of the process. I believed that I had been treated unfairly by Lovelace because to hire a foreigner a university has to be persuaded of this person's special merits. My initial performance had not been stellar, but it also seemed that my former colleagues had dramatically changed their minds about me before they found out who I really was and how my diversities could be an asset to them. I felt deleted like a nonentity whose existence does not count. I had considered suing them as a way to affirm my existence, and the opportunity arose when the position I had held was re-advertised and no one was hired.

To hire a foreign national, a university must demonstrate to the federal office of Immigration and Naturalization Services that this candidate is more qualified than any U.S. national who has applied. Understandably, the bar is higher for immigrants than it is for minorities who are U.S. nationals. I accepted this fact even though I was aware that the system conspired to have it result in pitting immigrants, who were noncitizens, against people of color, which is a disempowering situation for both parties. A hiring like mine, in an English department, could not have been based on the "nativism" that gets me hired in Italian, namely the presumed benefit of hiring "native speakers" to teach foreign language classes. It should have been based on the school's solid assessment of my competence as a candidate. And it could have been further justified by a genuine desire to diversify the background and cultural perspectives of a campus faculty, and the benefits for the educational process therein implied.

I believed in the plurality of knowledge, and in including those who help educational systems access it via their diverse backgrounds. In my mind, that desire for diversity, which had guided my journey to North America, was the ultimate purpose of equal opportunity employment and affirmative action. The case gave me a chance to see the misogyny and xenophobia that lurked behind the façade of that desire. Misogyny because I was a relatively young woman who had, solo, dared to think of herself as free to decide where and how to live her life. Xenophobia because I was not prepared to blend in and become one of the fold, by, say, forming a "family" based on the monogamous, heterosexist, and racially segregated rules of the local culture. Indeed, my only sexual partner in Netherville had been a black male immigrant from Muslim Africa. I am persuaded that in a more open climate my knowledge about drama, which had been so vehemently attacked, could have been more easily recognized. But I was still traversed by the transpersonal energies that fueled my resentment and sense of powerlessness, and not yet able to realize how problematic this recognition might have been at that time. My take on the subject matter took into account the influence of feminism, Deconstruction, and psychoanalysis, with a special attention to things Italian, and to reflect my longtime interest in vernacular cultures. The emphasis on theater as a communal art, which was on my mind, produced drama as a text distilled from that commonality, and my pedagogy placed the focus on the work of a theater ensemble rather than on individual actors and their stardom.

Going through the lawsuit process was crushing, especially because, for two years, I represented myself. While I learned to see myself with the eyes of those who had turned me down, I also had to learn all about the procedural part, which I did thanks to the advice of an attorney who generously helped me out. To begin with, as the suit started, the university barred any contacts between former colleagues and me. Embarrassed about my failure at Lovelace with almost everyone at Riverside, I now felt completely excluded from the academic world I had inhabited since the beginning of my life in the United States. My anxiety mounted. I was afraid I'd not make it and thought I was going nuts. Romina, the coordinator of Bi-Forum, gave me free individual psychotherapy sessions, and I went to the UCSD library to consult the DSM manual.

I called Romina. "Do you think I have bipolar disorder or something?"

"In your case," she said, "your syndrome could be diagnosed as post-traumatic stress disorder, which is what you get when you've fought in Vietnam."

Had I so wished, she was ready to diagnose me for disability benefits. But I called B. J. at UCR, and he strongly advised against it, because, he said, I would be sorry about it when I'd look for another job.

I became more immersed in my bisexual life. At the bi community parties, I was learning to enjoy amenities such as private pools and hot tubs. Soaking and skinny-dipping in good company were wonderful ways to socialize, and there were three houses fully equipped for the task. Romina had a large two-story house with an open downstairs floor plan, and a completely private backyard with pool and hot tub. Furry carpets and sofas made it especially comfortable. The kidney-shaped pool had a nice view of the city lights. The hot tub was under a white wooden canopy. Dave lived in an older neighborhood next to the Kearny Mesa canyons. His living room was decorated with batiks and figurines from the shadow theater in China. The lights were soft, and the dancing area filled up fast at the long-stroke sounds of new-age music. The backyard was a large garden leading to the top of the canyon. The Jacuzzi was out there, in the midst of trees and plants. Amanda lived in the North County inland area. Her house was a two-story, with thick carpets and a small yard. The hot tub had good jets and was next to the den, where people lay down after the bath.

It was a world of liquid effusions and spontaneous eroticism. Bodies became intimate and fused in a shared aura of magic sensuality. Potlucks were open to the whole community, and invitations announced at what time the party would become clothing optional. This gave everyone the opportunity to gradually experiment with new things without having anyone push their boundaries. People also exchanged hugs long and deep enough to feel the openness of their chakras. As our breathing rhythms became paced with one another, our spiritual energies and auras became one.

The Center, now called GLBT Center for inclusiveness, where our group now met also had psychotherapy programs staffed by interns. Identifying as a bisexual was an option, and so I signed up. My therapist, Linda, was a graduate student in a nearby university who had been a social worker and was making a career change. She tried to resurrect memories of sexual abuse from my father, and I insisted I had none. Then we got to Sara. I explained how close she was to her female friends, and that I had taken her to the Pride Festival.

"She's going to visit me again," I said. "I don't want to hide from her and don't want her judgment to dry up my vital energies."

"There's only one way," Linda explained, "and that's coming out to her."

We decided I would do this in a letter, which I wrote, one half in Italian and the other half in English, and mailed to her address. Giulio had moved back to Sardinia with her, and both were staying with his parents. The answer was devastating. "I do respect your choices, *Mamma*," Sara said, "but I'm not prepared to handle the situation." She canceled the trip she was about to take. To find comfort, she spent a weekend with Beatrice, Dario's lover, who later reported to me about how the two of them had wept together on the misfortune I brought upon them. At the time, I wondered if she had also confided in her dad.

A few months later, Dario and Beatrice came to visit me with my brother, Andrea. The occasion was Andrea's wedding, to be celebrated in London a few months later. But I now know that another reason was their anxiety about me, which might have caused some of their excessive drinking at the time. I was on the defensive and we spoke of nothing that mattered. They footed the bill and got to decide where we ate. We didn't have one single meal in a café, only wine-serving restaurants. I had about one-third of what they had to drink, and at the end of the week I was exhausted.

Andrea said, "*Papà* wants to talk to you. He wants to know what projects you have for your future."

I said I would, but in the morning, when he was somewhat sober. "There's no real conversation between a person under the influence and one that is not," I observed, "and I don't see why I should poison myself."

The conversation was very simple. I told Dario that I was doing what I needed to do to get well. "If you want to contribute," I said, "you're welcome." He agreed to partly fund my rent for a year or so. They left.

A few days later, I got a call from Giulio's sister-in-law.

"Gaia," she said, "I don't know if you're aware of this, but something is happening and I think you should know."

"What?" I said.

"Well, Sandra, you know she's been with Giulio for a long time now."

"Well?"

"Well, she's having a baby!" I thanked her and went to bed for four days. *How could this have happened without anybody telling me?* I reflected. I called Sara and asked.

"It's none of your business," she said.

"You bet it is my business. You're my daughter, and you're about to have a sister! Don't you think I should know?"

No reply.

I called Beatrice, who admitted to knowing about it, but that she didn't feel it was her place to tell me. "Why visit me, then?" I exclaimed.

But I had not told them what was new in my life, either. I faxed Dario, "As long as our relationships are so insincere," I wrote, "there's no point in my coming to the wedding." But then I realized I had kept something important from him just as he had.

"You don't have to come, but Andrea will be disappointed," Dario faxed back.

"There is something I can do to make our relationships better," I replied, "and that's telling you what's new and exciting in my life. I've been going out with women, *Papà,* and I love it!"

Dario answered, "Fine with me. We'll see to it all at the wedding."

He didn't have a heart attack, as Beatrice and Andrea feared. He was fine, maybe curious, an aspect of sexuality he had not explored in his erotic poetry and memoir. *I need someone to go with me now,* I reflected.

My neighbor Eileen was Irish American and she was just breaking up with her nine-year girlfriend. I asked her to accompany me. Sara was in such shock that she wouldn't spend a single hour alone with me. But by invoking patriarchal authority and getting my defiance accepted, I had at least shown her that who I was was okay. This was the beginning of a luminous friendship between my father and myself. My honesty was completely gratuitous, and with an idealist like Dario it could only pay off. I wrote Giulio and Sandra to congratulate them on their baby, telling them that if they needed a divorce, I'd be happy to oblige. A few months later, I flew to Rome, where I met Dario, who accompanied me to Sassari to sign the papers. The attorney asked, "Do you have any comments at this time, Ms. Cosentini?"

"Yes," I said, "when Sara was with me, she was a healthy baby. Now she's got a million ailments. I wonder why?" I turned to Giulio. "I think she's still a healthy child, and I want you to think about her that way as well."

Guilio promised he'd be more encouraging with her.

As I returned to San Diego, I became more and more involved with the Bi Forum group. At one point I realized I no longer owned any swim suits, for we went only to Blacks, the last nudist beach on the California shore. I also volunteered for the organization by coordinating phone calls to the membership the weekend before a monthly meeting. I remembered the call I received after my first meeting, and knew it mattered. A few months later, Romina, the coordinator, announced she needed a break. I volunteered, and with another woman, Vicky, we became co-coordinators. It was great to have a chance to give back to the community that saved my life. At home I struggled with pleadings and court orders, which reminded me of the past, but my social life was wonderful and I was living my bisexuality to the fullest. A whole world was opening up, and it had answers to what blocked my thinking in Netherville. My book benefited. Big chunks of text would pour out of me, and they would miraculously fill the gap between two previously written sections I had not been able to match.

Meanwhile, my suit was advancing, and a court date had been scheduled. I flew to Netherville one more time. My attorney told me all my ex-colleagues were rehearsing their parts with their attorneys, "'Cause you've given them the runs."

I was proud. I waited for my day in court. But the night before an order came out that dismissed the case. A twenty-four-page explanatory memorandum was attached to it. My attorney said, "A twelve-page memorandum is unusually long. This one is mammoth."

We examined the situation, and realized we could have taken on the challenge of taking the case to the next level. But despite my efforts to reach out to organizations such as the ACLU and the Women's Defense Fund, no one at that point had taken my case to heart. Perhaps it was not exemplary enough—or too difficult to fight. The case was taking about one-third of my time, and my money was running out. I knew that Lovelace had more power because it could stake out longer than I. So I agreed to give up and they agreed to pay their own attorneys. I realized the U.S. judicial system was a lot easier to activate than the Italian one, but not necessarily more effective in protecting the weak or creating more justice.

XI
Threesomes

The bisexual community I found in San Diego was the body that resurrected my buried lesbian self. As a second-wave feminist in the 1970s, I aimed for the goal of separating feelings from erotic pleasure. But the feelings would persist, and in the early 1990s I came to enjoy group sex partly as a way to reconnect feelings and erotic expression in a polyamorous way. I was in my late thirties, and learned to love all my lovers at the same time, together and separately, and to encourage each of them to love each other, with or without me, in the same way. It was a great liberation, for which, ironically, I have to thank the presumed AIDS epidemic. The fear of the fear of getting infected is what made safer sex necessary. Sexual players had to be open about their identities and practices. Everything had to be consensual, and risks were negotiated. Water-based lubricants, always at hand, replaced the body fluids that would not be exchanged. The erotic knowledge thus exchanged helped us find a healthy mode for our emotional, physical, and spiritual ways.

In my first encounters with women, a male body always acted as a willing and eager mediator; I would not have made it in any other way. In my erotic adventures with men, I had learned to suppress my feelings, but that was because my best friend, a girl, would listen to my confessions. To shield myself emotionally from men, a confidante was necessary. But the game in reverse just did not play. How could I trust that a woman could be as gullible as a man? Would I wound her in the same way? And who would be my confidante, should I be wounded in my own turn?

At my early bisexual parties I found myself among friends. These were not the conventional orgies of yore, in which a woman was presumed to be willing to do anything just because she was there. Nor was it a San Francisco bathhouse for gay men, where sex was supposedly turgid, anonymous, and fast-paced. The parties were usually organized by the long-standing members of the bi community, and were open to participants in Bi Forum, the local bi support and discussion group. The understanding was that what bisexuals needed most was a social space in which we could be ourselves, instead of passing as gay or straight. Founders and coordinators believed that just talking about coming-out issues in the context of support-group meetings was not sufficient to create it. They encouraged older group members to open up their homes to newer members, who were thus invited to parties and socials based on rules established by the hosts.

The preferred homes were equipped with warm, bubbling hot tubs conducive of group ablutions and soaking, and large, carpeted, barely furnished living rooms open for play. The floor was open for group hugs, fondling, necking, and the kind of gentle massage and intimate conversation that at times evolved into more. It was an atmosphere of inclusiveness and acceptance, where people of many colors, ages, and shapes gradually learned to surrender their sense of fear and shame, to feel confident that their boundaries would be respected, and to play out the erotic scenarios they fantasized about. The AIDS era made safety an imperative. But precisely because we had chosen a flamboyantly sex-positive posture, we needed to be sure that exchanges of fluids were consensual, and that a participant's personal integrity was respected. Those of us who were somewhat in charge of the organization made sure that people who showed up at parties had an adequate support-group experience—that no flippant intruder would spoil the game. Precisely because all action and the very fabric of the community were designed to promote healthy and pleasurable modes of sexual expression, no substances were used, not even pot, and there was barely any alcohol. All of the sexual and erotic energy came from the group's effort to be present to our partners and friends, to honor their erotic imagination, and to be open to giving and receiving the gifts of love and pleasure that were freely circulated.

My first threesome was with a male Russian émigré from Georgia, and a female émigré from France. Lev was dark and handsome, with marked features, and thick body hair in black curls. Marguerite was petite, with a cute Parisian nose, light brown hair, and beautiful round tits with pointy nipples. We were at Dave's, and the hot tub was at the end of the large rear garden, its path marked by a line of candles in sand-filled brown bags, up to the deck on top of the canyon slope. The city lights were far away, the air was chilly, the vegetation fragrant. The water was a bit too warm for my taste, but it gradually cooled off as the night grew younger. It was a concrete Jacuzzi, about five feet in diameter, three deep. All around the bottom circumference was a step for our sweet buns to rest on.

People arrived to the platform in the nude, and hung their towels on the railing. Each body had a special kind of beauty; every body was lovable; breasts resting comfortably on a woman's stomach; men with slim legs and thin hair; white, mushy flesh, birthmarks, freckles, shades of olive and ebony; indulgent doughnuts and protruding potbellies. The ugly and the handsome rubbed elbows and their auras became one. Big lesson for those caught up in the lookist culture emanating from Hollywood. In the tub, people talked about poetry, literature, some movie, or culture and politics. A young man tried to pick an argument, but it was hard to fight in that kind of setting. The discussion was stimulating but not argumentative. In that magic setting, words easily melted into soft strokes as a player fondled another's foot, and talking went on. Eventually, another player came along, and found a space in the warm water. When the seat was full, new players sat on somebody else's lap.

"The more people in the Jacuzzi, the more room there is," Dave said philosophically as he lay next to a handsome black guy, "so many laps to sit on!" They fondled each other and kissed in a loving way as their skin colors melted in the moonlight shades. They were enjoying each other as their tender motions were being observed. It was one of the most beautiful scenes I ever saw!

The night of my first threesome the Jacuzzi was not very full, and we kind of ran the show. Marguerite was sitting next to me, and on her other side was Lev. He was fondling her breast, and I noticed that she did not mind my watching. I extended my hand and touched her other breast. She seemed to enjoy. It was the first time I touched a woman's breast erotically. It was so wonderful! I did not know why, I could not imagine how I had waited so long. I noticed with joy that Lev accepted my intrusion and welcomed it. The erotic energy grew

stronger in the field between the three of us. Marguerite smiled bliss-
fully as our fondling hands moved on to touch her waist and abdomen, and then her legs and feet. We massaged her sweetly and
tenderly, as in a concerted dance, while our two bodies had not directly touched yet. Lev was very erotic, but at that point, an unmedi-
ated, direct contact with a male of such sexual prowess would have
been too threatening for me. The presence of Marguerite's sweeter
and gentler person made me feel at home. Eventually, we left the tub
area and returned to the living room where the rest of the party was.
It must have been late.

The party was tapering off. Perhaps other sexual activities were going on in the various bedrooms, but we were not sure. We were aware
of the host's generosity to the bisexual community, of his commitment to favoring its expression. Before retiring to his bedroom, Dave
made sure we had enough lube and condoms. We lay on the sofa. Lev
was between Marguerite and myself. We were all very wet and horny.
His arms extended on opposite sides, as his hands moved toward our
respective Mons Veneris, and his fingers gradually opened up our labia. He was being fair and generous. Marguerite and I occasionally
looked at each other and smiled. Our arms touched behind his back.
The excitement was growing, as our vulvas became wet and his fingers kept fondling our outer genitals. It was great to hear another
woman's heavy breathing, imagine what was going on in there just as
my breathing was accelerating also. Lev, I bet, was feeling very proud
of himself. But I believe he knew he was not the only source of that
kind of erotic energy. The odor of soaked skin swishy and wet with
bodily juices enveloped the three of us in a collective aura. Eventually,
Lev lay down on the sofa on his back, his cock erect. Marguerite put a
condom on it, and kneeled over his crotch.

She started to ride him, and I thought for a moment, *Well, maybe
this is the right time for me to withdraw* . . . but I held Marguerite's hand,
and she held on to mine, so I stayed. It was exciting to feel so close to
their erotic energy, as if my body was a vehicle for it also. The heavy
breathing became faster, until Marguerite brazenly came. But Lev
was still holding. I had rarely seen a male lover with such control. His
cock obeyed him perfectly. He was on a high plateau of ecstasy, but

had not expended himself yet. Well, Marguerite was off him, his cock was still hard, and we had another condom. So I put it on the rod, and started my own ride. Marguerite stayed near me while I rode and rode until my orgasm came, at which point Lev came also. Eventually, we resumed our positions on the sofa. The air was still thick with erotic energy. We all had expended ourselves, but the game was so exciting that it had produced more excitement in the process. Eventually, Lev and Marguerite started to play doggy style. The breathing became heavier and louder. I enjoyed watching them from close by, being there to feel their excitement. I used to love the style myself, and seeing another woman enjoying made me feel happy.

When they came the three of us were still enveloped in our dense aura of erotic energy. I had returned to a peripheral position with respect to the two other players, like the one in which I started. It was maybe 4 a.m. as the excitement gradually dissolved and we came back to our senses. Each one of us started to look for his or her belongings and clothes, until we finally got our stuff together and prepared to take off. We could have stayed overnight, but evidently we each preferred to sleep in our own bed. We were a little confused as we parted. Perhaps each one of us had done something really new and transforming. Just as our erotic communication had happened primarily through our bodies, so our leave-taking was also nonverbal. We simply gave each other a long, warm group hug and walked outside, each to our own car, with smiling faces full of longing and happiness. We had not decided that we would repeat the experience or meet again. In fact, I was still new enough to the group, I wasn't sure I remembered their names. Eventually, we met at several other parties, and became more acquainted with each other in a nonsexual way, but that miracle did not repeat itself in the same way.

The next stage of development came at one of Amanda's parties, during group sex with me at the center of a powerful erotic wave. Amanda was in her forties and ill with chemical sensitivities which had prompted a career change, from chemist to naturopath. She was writing a book like myself. It was our first, and we used to have cautiously encouraging conversations on the topic. Her book was on natural health and medicine. Amanda was a very calm person—her affect somewhat low—but she was resilient and determined. Her skin was pale, and her graying hair flew in large waves down to her neck. Her body showed moderate signs of aging in a proud, handsome way, with her wide hips, her large breasts gracefully resting on her upper abdomen, and her low muscular tone. She looked like an erotic mother and fertility goddess.

The party started in the living room, and then gradually moved into the backyard, where the hot tub was located, and then finally into the den. Floors were covered with soft, furry carpets in blue tones, and walls were decorated with silky fabrics in purple and orange. The den was equipped with a fireplace and a stereo. The ceiling's triangular shape was lined with a batik fabric softly pinned up from its center and corner, with its geometrical design gently flowing down in a round curve.

The new age music filled up the space with its liquid sounds and long strokes. Loreena McKennitt and Enja were my all-time favorites. The den and the hot tub were fairly close to one another, and the interior space was rather open, so that the sound of the music circulated and wrapped us up in its aura. Amanda liked to give parties, and was fairly successful in having fun in them. She lay down almost motionless, while several lovers pleasured her by gently touching her body and genitals, as her soft moans exuded her secretive joy. Watching her enjoyment was an encouragement for all her guests to also participate.

Amanda's hot tub was a large dark green, made of plastic in a square shape, with strong water jets placed above the curved seats. People got in and out of its hot water, an ideal place to warm up for the den, where most of the action happened. Players came in from the backyard door in groups of two or three, wrapped in their towels or holding them in their hands. They laid the towels on the carpet and lay down over them, forming cozy little niches as they arranged them. From the stereo the music spread resonating throughout the triangular space. The ceiling decoration evoked the sky and infused a sense of serenity. Players smelled the odorous bodies softened by the warm water. They used their towels to dry each other's bodies, and then from drying they moved on to exchanging soft strokes, and then more fondling, and caressing a person's hair and curls.

Players looked into each other's eyes and talked softly, "How does this feel?"

"Could you please massage my ankle?"

"I love your hair."

"Your skin feels wonderful."

"May I fondle your breasts?"

More players left the hot tub area and moved into the den. The floor would be covered with towels and with soft, moistened bodies lying down with each other in various shapes and combinations. The motions were slow and graceful, as players nested next to each other according to the erotic energy emanating from their bodies and auras. Each individual aura gradually amalgamated with other auras, as neighboring players got closer to each other and their energetic bodies became more connected. The sexual energy circulated freely from person to person, and with no obstacles present, its intensity multiplied by the number of players involved. The erotic energy traversed the triangular ocean of bodies in motion like a wave; it was attracted toward an area of more intense play. Then the nearby areas became more quiet, as players turned to the nearby focus, and contributed to its intensity with their admiring gaze. Motion and contemplation alternated in an ebb and flow of erotic waves. Seeing others in a love embrace was being part of the show, since all players were present to each other and contributing energy to the erotic game.

Men were tender to each other like babies. Women touched in a reverent, almost religious way. All kinds of combinations were displayed: in one corner, two middle-aged women and a younger man fondled and caressed in a loving way; in another corner, two young men looked into each other's eyes tenderly; a little further, a man and a woman leaned against each other and touched each other's genitals; next to the fireplace, two young women stroked each other's hair and fondled each other's breasts; another couple simply sat and watched while holding each other's hand. The kinds of people that participated were different also. Male-female couples in their fifties had been part of this scene for much longer than the young men who just barely joined. Some players were in great physical shape and their trim bodies made a handsome display. Others bodies were as wide as oceans, with overflowing limbs and flesh whose abundance made its own kind of charming display. Our organization reached out to a diverse population, even as whites were a majority. But diversity at our events contrasted with its academic variety. There it was forced as in a zoo, with everyone as a specimen. Our players represented the fabric of American society in a more genuine way. They were thin or fat, silky or hairy, masculine or feminine, pale or olive, dark or blond, successful or depressed, well-off or broke, college-educated or self-taught, short or tall. But they were all lovable for they were here to be with others like them. Here I could touch the erotic energy their auras emanated, and realized it was the same energy that, invisible, animates inadvertent players when social conventions operate.

Paul had introduced me to the Bi-Forum and he was manning the organization's booth when I went to my first Gay Pride Festival. Surely I had been attracted to that booth by some magnetic energy. Like me, he had moved to the United States for a research project, which fell through. He was soft and cozy, and had that European effeminacy I usually like in men. A French Jew from Algeria, he had returned to France after the independence war, and landed in California eventually. In the Bi-Forum group he found a community and a family. He was also an animator, and made a tremendous effort to reeducate himself to our community's inclusive, spiritual, and polyamorous ways. When I joined the group, he tried to establish a one-on-one relationship with me, which, as I pointed out, was not what I needed at the time, and ran against the grain of our vision. He was a perfectly reliable male lover who could keep his erection indefinitely. He was not as good-looking as Lev, but more artistic and sensitive. I had been one of five women surrounding him in a group love embrace, which really facilitated my approach to a woman's body, my acceptance of the erotic energy therein contained.

At Amanda's party we were neighbors on the den's carpet floor. At one point the group-sex wave came toward our area, and those around us felt that some strong chemistry was present in the energy field between us. The intimacy and confidence we had established both physically and intellectually paid off. Eventually, I found myself on top of him, and the ride began. The erotic energy of the whole group became focused on our performance. It became the central point of the orgy and the leading force of the wave. As I was on top, I became the focal point of the group-sex event, and the erotic intensity multiplied for us by the number of persons in the group, as it also multiplied for everybody else. It felt great, and I wondered why I had always had sex behind closed doors before. I felt completely absorbed by this genuine and authentic expression of eroticism.

As the party tapered off and people started to go home, I also eventually left and went to sleep in my own bed, as I usually preferred. I pleasured myself a little before going to sleep, as I usually did after a party. I hadn't exchanged fluids and so some clitoral, labial, vaginal, or anal area that had been stimulated in group-sex had not been properly taken care of just yet. So as to have a good night's sleep I took care of it myself and went to sleep. At that time, the dream of forgiveness came. I was in bed with Stephane and his wife. He was the lover of six years who left me for another woman, returned to Europe, and abandoned me to my American destiny. She was the woman I had been deadly jealous of, who stole my love and benefited from all the lessons I had given him; the woman I wanted to seduce away from him, to show her how fickle his love was. In my dream, she was with us sharing our bed. My jealousy evaporated. She was soft and loving. He was on one side and she was on the other. They embraced me and held me, they felt my pain, the pain of abandonment that their union and happiness cost me, and they embraced my chest to heal that pain. In the dream fantasy, the two objects of my desire were together and they were with me as well. I felt love for both of them equally, and I forgave them. It was the compersion effect, as I learned later on. All of a sudden, their decision to be together without me was not a rejection, but simply a result of the social conventions of monogamy. In a polyamorous world, we could all have loved each other profusely, and we surely would, since we the two women in the triad shared our love for the man. I felt an integral part of their erotic energy, a force that had contributed to their coming together, and had done so in spite of myself. Now my contribution was acknowledged and I could feel proud to have made them happy in my own way.

XII
Awareness

North County is about thirty minutes north of downtown San Diego, between La Jolla, where the UCSD campus is located, and the navy base of Oceanside, toward LA. The coastal area is studded with beach towns in the style of the French Riviera, complete with chic shopping centers, stylish boutiques, and classy restaurants. But as one drives north, it becomes more casual. Cardiff is a surfers' village between 101, the Coastal Highway, and Five, the Freeway. Its few rows of decked houses with small yards are perched on a steep slope overlooking a wavy ocean area.

Hippies and other new age types populate the area, their lives as unplanned as those of habitués at Miracles, the local café. A few more hang-outs line the coastal highway, up to the ashram of the Self-Realization Fellowship, with its meditation gardens on the sea point. Then there is Encinitas, with its health food restaurants, artisan shops, and metaphysical bookstores. The colorful flyers posted to ubiquitous advertising boards speak of a community bursting with energy. Neo-pagan firewalks, moonlight Wicca rituals, discounted massage sessions, biofeedback, guided meditation, all kinds of new holistic-health methods are the kinds of activities one can get involved in. The whole area is very environmentally conscious, with recycling at the curb and fresh produce available from nearby organic farms. The area around the ashram teems with healers in various specialties, including chiropractic, Reiki, bodywork, colonics, acupuncture, nutrition, homeopathy, and natural gynecological care. The Sunday market smells of incense and sage, with wind chimes dangling from the stands, and new age CDs on vendors' boom-boxes. It is there that I healed from the diseases of modernity. The sense of holism I learned made the magic of contemplation and meditation accessible.

When I finished *The "Weak" Subject,* I realized I had terrible arthritis and back pains. *What can I do?* I thought to myself. I was reluctant to take medicines, for my health insurance was very basic and I was living on my savings. A local woman came to my door and told me about Super Blue-Green Algae, a food supplement she recommended. It was rather expensive but I decided to try it anyway. I read all the literature and it seemed persuasive. The problem was the foods we eat are contaminated with antibiotics, pesticides, and steroids, they explained. The pains are a result of toxicity stored in the body. This wild food would reactivate my system and infuse it with new energy. It came from soil near a volcanic lake, rich with minerals and other nutritive elements and it was a microorganism easy to absorb. Exercise was recommended, and I started doing more of it.

"Keep at it," the woman said. "Remember, it's a food, not a medicine. As it enters your system, your metabolism will gradually change. If it makes you feel dizzy or strange, it's because you're responding to it. It means you need even more."

The algae really gave me new energy and I stayed on it. But still, metacarpal tunnel on my right wrist would not go away and I was wearing a brace. I thought of getting massage, but how many sessions would I need before I felt better? A couple of massage schools were in the vicinity, and I longed to be in some kind of organized activity. *Wouldn't it be better to take a course in massage instead?* I told myself. So I enrolled at Vitality Training Center (VTC) and came home to a whole different way of learning. There, the body was not an abstraction, it was mass, flesh. And touching it was not appropriating it in some perverse way; it was healing it, giving it back to itself. There were no mind games, and one didn't have to be guarded against them, so that one could practice trust and sharing. Of the 100 hours of course time, about half was spent working on a fellow student's body, the other half having one's body worked on. Of course, a teacher's guidance was essential, and VTC teachers were very generous with their knowledge, giving us an inclusive perspective on the field of holistic health, with massage as the center in a whole spectrum of possible therapies. My back turned out to be an asset to the course. It had all kinds of problems: spasms, sublaxations, knots, tense nerves. The teacher worked on it until it became smooth like the Pacific. It was wonderful, and I was happy that my investment paid so well.

I was still finishing the course, when I heard that a massage facility in Oceanside was looking for therapists. The clientele was military, but the place was "clean," no hand jobs or other sexual requests. Licensing is heavily regulated in California, and the police crack down on places that don't abide by the law. The owner was an honest guy with modest aspirations. An infinite supply of customers was at hand, and he wanted to play it safe. He only hired "girls" that would not get around the rules and make an extra buck. The work was on commission, 50 percent plus tips. I showed up and was hired. I started to work, and still remember my first massage, when I had learned only arms and torso. I did it with such joy and fervor that the guy didn't notice. The clientele was not very sophisticated but there were many nice fellows, mostly young Marines who told stories about Okinawa and other faraway destinations. Fear and loneliness prevailed. They did fantasize about sex, but were open to the proposition that massage was great, that it could relax their hamstrings and sacrum, all the while infusing their system with new energy and making their bodies feel whole again. They got it that it was better than a meager hand job, something they could do for free on their own.

I got along with other massage therapists. Competition was not encouraged, even though being "requested" by a client was a plus. A young woman from Russia was very distinguished and good mannered. She did very well working to support herself as a student at the nearby university, Cal State San Marcos. When she learned I had a PhD, she asked me many questions on graduate education in the United States. I couldn't give her a positive assessment, since I felt the system had betrayed me. It was a time when retiring professors were being replaced by adjuncts, paid by the course, and hired a day or two before the beginning of each semester with no retirement or health benefits. To make things worse, universities continued to churn out PhDs, so as to irresponsibly saturate the market even more.

"What hope is there in the profession? It's better to be a massage therapist," I told her. But still, she was an achiever and my failure could not discourage her.

I made my own flyer and posted it to the boards in the hang-outs that lined the coastal area. People started to call and I dressed my extra bedroom with a futon and a massage table. When the first clients came, I breathed deeply and projected confidence and professionalism. No accident ever happened. The clients I was getting were better; they had more experience with massage and responded more articulately to my methods. I called my massage "holistic" because it was a combination of techniques, Swedish, Shiatsu, sports massage, and Reiki. Also, it was a way to facilitate a client's awareness of his or her body as an organic, interconnected whole. Trust and a chosen passivity were of the essence. I was learning to read the body like an open book, a text that spoke to me of its stored problems and tensions.

It was not long before Julie contacted me, a massage therapist from Encinitas who had her practice at the North County Healing Arts Center. "Are you interested in renting a massage space?" she asked. "The overhead is low; you'd be sharing with me."

I thought about it, and wasn't sure I was ready. But then, continuing at home was dangerous. I did not have the qualifications for a license to practice independently, and the Center offered the supervision of practitioners who did. I went for it. The Healing Arts Center was a magical place, with its serene, terse air, metaphysical decorations, narrow corridor, and vanilla walls. Affirmations and holistic principles were on display. "We're not just here to make a living; we're here to make a difference," one poster proclaimed. Another said, "Disease is the body screaming for attention." Our massage room smelled of wild sage. Wreaths and framed icons decorated the walls. The light in from the long window on the corner made the decorations glow. As I opened my own business, I prepared an even better flyer for myself, with my picture and a logo from a pair of sculpted hands by Auguste Rodin. My face was now on all the local advertising boards. The business did well from the start and I gradually made regular clients, whose progress I could observe. It felt great! Many of them really got over major hurdles; their lives took interesting new turns. Each body told a story it was my privilege to interpret; each spoke to me in its own language, my hands responding to its requests with the appropriate touch, sequence of strokes, and pressure. I realized these clients trusted me completely, and that was empowering to them. They lay in front of me naked on their bellies, completely defenseless. Their surrender, the chosen passivity they gifted to themselves, was the beginning of their regeneration process.

I had finished the research project for which I came to the San Diego area, even as the book was late to come out for I hadn't found a publisher yet. I had a successful business, nice friends. My life was pulling itself together after all. *It's time to be the hostess for a Bi Forum party,* I thought to myself. I didn't have a hot tub or a pool, but I did have a massage room cum table, a nice deck over the roof, and a large living room with ocean view. I decided to open my home. The invitation flyer announced a potluck party, clothing-optional after 10 p.m., with massage room available. It was a great party and lots of people came, including players from the Family Synergy group, who were bi swingers with family. They traveled with kids, who went to sleep wherever. After the party, I remember finding a five- and an eight-year-old in my bed. It was 6 a.m. and I had to get some sleep for I had to work the next day.

The evening started slow, with people from different groups getting acquainted. At around 10 p.m. the nonnudist types went home and the others started to get comfortable. The Synergy group had some professional dancers who improvised a beautiful seduction ritual performed at the rhythm of a Native American dance. The dancers had handsome, healthy bodies adorned with Indian embellishments and engaged each other from opposite ends of the living room, thus wrapping everyone in their wave of erotic energy.

At about eleven, Eliza came. She was with Sasha, her partner from Russia, and lived in LA. Eliza had been married twice and had two girls. She had been an activist in Central America and worked in the Evening School District of LA. She smelled like jasmine and roses, with wide green eyes, a light-olive skin, and a regular, oval face. Her ash-brown hair was long and curly; it had a life of its own and was always somewhat rebellious. Her body was trim and delicate, with thin bones and long legs. She was capable of the most powerful orgasms I'd seen or heard of. The massage room started to fill up. When I got there, a bit late for I'd been playing hostess, the massage table and the futon were taken. Amanda was on the table, with somebody massaging her. Sasha and Eliza were on the futon and I joined them. I had made love with them before, and knew it was some of the best. I enjoyed being with both, and they did as well. It wasn't machismo or jealousy. Sasha was the most unpossessive of lovers, having agreed that Eliza visit me alone for a whole weekend on a previous occasion. But without him it just wasn't the same. Nor was his presence intrusive at all for he liked to watch women make love so well it was a pleasure to have him there. It was not impotence on his part for he was a very good lover himself. This evening they were together when I entered and was invited to join them. We did it in a lot of different shapes, the triangle forever transforming and flowing with energy. Eventually, the party tapered off and just a few people stayed.

Eliza and Sasha were spending the night, since they had driven from LA. They had some videos with them, and said, "You have to watch this, Gaia." They knew I was a safer-sex educator, and wanted me to become alert to the fact that not everybody agreed on where AIDS came from. It was about 3 a.m. and they played HEAL tapes with investigative journalist Jon Rappaport and virologist Peter Duesberg, from U.C. Berkeley. I listened, amazed, at what they were saying.

That AIDS science was a scam invented to control people's sexuality and health; that it was political and there was nothing scientific or objective to it. That there wasn't, and had never been any infectious epidemic: the numbers just weren't there, but the public was not told because authorities thought they'd fuck like rabbits if they were informed. That we had been duped to believe that what usually meant you were safe, testing positive for antibodies, now meant the opposite—that you were infected. That there was a reason why the promised vaccine never came: there never was an infectious virus to begin with. That the proclaimed discovery of 1984 was a political ploy to get Reagan reelected, a press conference held at the high point of the campaign. That it was plagiarism, since the virus had been stolen from the Pasteur Institute in France. That Robert Gallo, the "discoverer," had patented the test the very same day. That big pharmaceutical companies, like Glaxo Wellcome, were making money from selling "cures" that were more poisonous than the disease itself; waging fear into those allegedly at risk. That the collapse of one's immune system, deployed in various forms, including cancer, multiple sclerosis, and AIDS itself, was nothing but the end result of generalized environmental deterioration.

Especially when in combination with excessive stress and use of drugs, contamination of air, food, and water could do the trick without any infectious agent, the dissenters claimed. How sensible! Duesberg was a serious scientist from the Max Planck Institute in Berlin and then Berkeley, but he had lost all his grant money for he refused to play the game. His laboratory was closed, and he was back to teaching Science 101 to undergrads, when he finally decided to go public and denounce the Centers for Disease Control and other grant agencies. The tapes were compiled by a volunteer community organization based in LA called HEAL (Health Education Alliance Liaison). Institutions had gulped down all dissent space!

At around 6 a.m. Eliza and Sasha left. I thanked them for their tapes and we promised we'd soon get back together. I was left with a new world in my imagination. How could I have been duped so well? When had I stopped asking questions? For the next two nights I did not sleep a wink. *Then, all my pains, losses, disappointments, and those of others, have been for nothing!* I thought to myself. There was no menace other than the fear we harbored within ourselves. And my environmentalist friends at Riverside had been right to predict that sooner than later the price of modernity would become too expensive even for those on top of the pyramid scheme that modern knowledge was.

I knew what was happening in the humanities, and, with the edifice of modern knowledge being based on science, I should not have been surprised that the same things were happening on the other side of the aisle, on a much bigger, more dangerous scale. Up to the mid-1980s, environmental studies were believed to hold the promise of a better future for both humankind and the planet. But since that time, in academic discourse they had become somewhat secondary, even as an environmental movement was on the rise in many areas of the country, with its spirituality, folklore, and sustainable practices such as vegetarianism, holistic health, and recycling. Of course, environmental awareness did not reach all of those who had been exposed to ecological hazards enough to damage their immune system in a serious way. Yet initially, many hypotheses were open to possibly explain why so many gay men who frequented the San Francisco bathhouses came down with severe immunosuppression and were hospitalized for the diseases that ensued. Many knew they ingested high amounts of medical and recreational drugs, while conducting highly stressful lives with little rest and much exchange of fluids with numerous partners, countless at times. A rush to discount the possibility of contagion was only natural at first. But why ban further investigation on any other possible cause just because a virologist with a questionable reputation proclaimed victory for himself? Virology had evidently its own war to wage.

Indeed, as I realized from the HEAL tapes, the focus on the infectious hypothesis is but a reflection of the way in which Western epistemology operates. Virology is an established field that can be easily fenced and appropriated. Its object is clear-cut: viruses and nothing but them. Virologists have an investment in demonstrating that viruses cause problems. Looking for causes in the ecological imbalances we have in our bodies is a way to approach the problem from a holistic perspective, and that's what thinkers steeped in Western epistemology are least adept in. Holistic knowledge is based on careful, delicate observation. Respectful of the integrity of the phenomenon it observes, it studies its objects in context, as elements in the ecosystem they are part of. Western epistemology claims to cure the diseases of modernity while in many cases it only promotes the mentality that causes them, as is the case with the AIDS scare. Holistic knowledge, on the other hand, promotes a gaian awareness, a sense of our planet as a living being we are part of, and this helps to generate the symbiotic reason that will make health scares unnecessary.

XIII
Body of Water

I decided to get myself to a lesbian party in nearby Rancho Santa Fe, a plush area with green hills and beautifully designed family homes. The town prided itself in liberalism so that, if wealthy enough, all kinds of couples were welcome. The party was at Georgia's, a stockbroker whose home was in a little bowl, with eucalyptus and palm trees, and a dirt road to the stable. Georgia and her lover loved horses, and one could visit their thoroughbreds down the road. It was nice for once to be among women, in a party where people wore clothes. Much as I liked the Bi Forum socialization, I longed for a women-only space, perhaps because I was concerned about Sara and my relationship with her. Eliza, who had two girls, was a present parent, boxed in this responsibility that overruled everything else. I, on the other hand, was an "absent parent," feeling excluded from my girl's progress into adulthood, unable to influence her. Lesbians knew what it felt like to be a rejected parent, for many would come out after they had babies, and would lose them in the process, like myself. Raising daughters to accept their mother's queerness proved especially difficult, since pressures to conform for acceptance were stronger on teen-age girls.

I arrived at the party and felt a bit out of place, a foreigner with no assets in such an affluent milieu. But people were friendly and a woman walked up to me and we struck up a conversation. She was heavy, with large breasts hanging from her wide shoulders, and overflowing hips and belly. About my height, she had round green eyes, a glowing smile and wavy red hair. "I am Emily," she said in a husky, sexy voice. She was full of questions, curious about my life and origins, and happily surprised that I would pay attention to her. We discovered both of us lived in Cardiff. Her architectural design studio was a couple of blocks down the road from my place. "That's where I spend my best days, doing what I love, designing luxury homes. My family lives in El Cajon, southeast San Diego. I have two boys and one girl, all of high school age and see them on weekends," she explained. Her majestic body spoke of a past beauty, its force stronger with its own memory.

After the party we had ice cream at a parlor in the area, and sat on the nearby bench for hours, talking about our semidissolved marriages, our relationships with our quasi-exes, our children, and their reactions to our coming out as gay women, and to our professional ambitions before that as well. It was wonderful to finally share my pain at feeling so discouraged by my family about my professional aspirations. Finally someone who understood the heaviness of a husband, ex or not, who feels that your self-improvement is his loss, for he can no longer dominate you. Finally someone who was rejected by her family for being honest with them. Finally someone who was a lesbian neither because men didn't like her nor because she didn't like them, but rather because she felt bonding with women was necessary, even erotically, to have the self-esteem and determination one needs for success. Finally someone who became a lesbian to make the world better and freer for her daughter, and was hoping she'd understand that some day.

Emily came to my place that evening and we embraced. I sat on the futon near the wood-covered wall, and she faced me. She took her top off, and her overflowing bosom filled up the space between us. There was a sweet smell to her hair and face, even though her expression at times betrayed the harshness she knew. Her breasts were wrapped in a large bra down to her waist, their flesh was soft and sensitive. I buried my face in the cleavage, and breathed deeply as in a trance. I told her I loved fat people, lovers one could touch profusely and with benefit. She seemed surprised but noted it is not uncommon for people to feel erotically attracted to fatness. "What is more difficult," she said, "is for people to accept you as a partner and a person."

We spent a long time in our love embrace before she attempted to go farther.

"Can we leave that for next time we get together?" I asked. And we did so.

Emily's condo was decorated with the most extravagant adornments, prevalent styles including Mexican, Southwestern, and California baroque. Every little corner had a life of its own, with stones, amulets, Indian pots, dried flowers, mirrors, stars, and sun shapes. Her favorite materials were wood and clay in a variety of textures and shades, earth tones mixed with green and an occasional blue or purple. The windows looked over the shore, and one could see the long Pacific waves curl up like white flames. The walls exhibited her history as an architect of designer homes, and as a one-time stunning beauty. Her home designs were in Spanish style, with arches, patios, tile roofs, and French doors, their expanded white bodies lined with red trim and surrounded with luxuriant plants. Her pictures portrayed her with her family, always in a midchest frame, her rough skin made silky with the studio's retouched negative. Her fantasy world was on display, and the fantasy magically corresponded to the reality of her creations.

The view from her upstairs bedroom was even more stunning, with a wider perspective on the northern San Diego bay. The bed, positioned sideways, was topped with a maplewood canopy, a lace band wrapped around it in wide circles, a hanging peg with a flannel parrot perched on it. The first time we made love, she promised to teach me everything she knew about women's eroticism, but she would not disrobe.

I said, "This doesn't work for me. I can't have sex with a person whose body I don't know."

She understood, and next time used a veil to cover the bumpy scar over her overflowing belly.

"I've had several operations," she explained. "I was about to die. They could not figure out what it was. That's why they fixed it so badly."

Emily was a generous lover. She had been an English teacher at one point, and loved to share her knowledge with good students. Her lessons were a delight in themselves, and proved very helpful later on. She loved a woman's body, and spent hours discovering sites of pleasure in my body I was hardly aware of. She also taught me how to use dildos and vibrators, a huge collection hidden in the corner behind the slanted bed. We discussed the AIDS scare. She was not too concerned, but since I wanted an open relationship with her, I felt responsible for protecting her. We decided to become primary partners and exchange fluids only among ourselves. We shared her toys and she showed me how to have fun with them. She tried a smooth one in my vagina and a rippled one in my anus. She also had a soft porn collection with mellow flicks in earth tones, women disrobing in front of a mirror, giving pleasure to themselves. She knew so much about women's pleasure. She noticed my clit was not too sensitive, and said, "It will improve with use, you know," and spent hours pressing her tongue against it as softly as I asked her.

Our past love stories became part of our erotic games for we were lovers and confidantes as well; a dream come true for me, as if both my high school best friend Emanuela and my graduate-school friend Geraldine had finally fallen in my bed. Emily listened to my stories about lovers, break ups, dreams, art, and pleasure. Sometimes she'd ask me to bring some pictures, and I did. I showed her Stephane and Sara, our little life in Riverside in the early 1980s. She felt curious and cozy. She accepted that I was bisexual, even though she continued to prefer the label lesbian for herself. Her husband was a professor, and she told me about her years as a wife, with her husband's colleagues making passes at her. Her fantasies about women, and her secret forays into the sex-industry world. Her gaining weight as a way to protect herself emotionally, and her having more peace as her looks faded away.

"Finally," she said, "the time for me to come out arrived. Lisa, a woman with whom I had had sex once in college, reappeared in my life, and I proposed to her. The relationship of my dreams began. But my family was in shock and made Lisa's life unbearable."

They broke up, and Emily was still thinking about her. "You look like Lisa," she said. "That's why I want to be with you."

I was very happy to fill this void, even though I sometimes felt Emily was a bit obsessed with her so I told her about the wonderful adventures I had in the bi community and invited her to share in them. She occasionally joined the parties, and once had sex with Lev. We talked about all our fantasies and adventures, never any jealousy entering our world. Indeed, those tales excited us even more, which made for better sex.

With Emily I learned to indulge my clit to a fault, her tongue soft, almost imperceptible, on my hood for hours, my mind spinning in ecstasy. I learned to love and admire my body and accept her admiration for it. Her eyes on my hips and her voice saying, "I love this curve. It's just so pretty. I could spend hours watching it." I learned to make love like an artist, enjoying every moment of our creation, and separating my pleasure from hers. Her wide labia open, my fingers in her birth canal, her clit getting moist and turgid. I learned to enjoy giving a woman an orgasm—feeling her body vibrate as she entered her fantasy world, her breathing dense as she squealed and came. Her body, like an ocean, overwhelmed me when I climbed over her belly and buried my head in her chest. Her breasts and abdomen were soft and yielding; liquid flesh like amniotic fluid or the immensity of a mother's bosom to a suckling baby; a generous mother whose womb one would want to enter again; the body of water all creatures come from.

Our relationship was like an eternal courtship in which we discussed being queer mothers of girls. Emily and I met at a time when each of us was negotiating a space independent from our respective families, while at the same time wanting to participate in our children's education. For her, it was creating a life around her architectural design studio, a life that supported her love for her job and the creativeness it involved. For me, it was creating a life around my efforts to finish my first book of research on women and modernity. For her, it was getting accepted as a mother who was also gay, and could model inclusiveness and acceptance for her children as well. For me, it was creating acceptance for me as a model of development in my family, one that Sara could look up to and respect as well. We were perfect for each other in many respects. I helped her see the model in herself, and she helped me. I told her about my grief over my daughter's rejection, first when she would not return to the United States, then when she canceled her trip after my coming-out letter. She told me all about her children's almost disgusted aloofness from her, when they learned about her first girlfriend. We spent long hours on the phone sorting things out, reasoning with one another, "Why would this be? How could this be explained?" As persons who traveled back and forth between the straight world of our families and the gay world of our relationship, we certainly knew a lot about homophobia as a governing taboo of Western families, second perhaps only to incest. We cherished our evenings together and valued our romance. We loved our periodic dates, quality time we dedicated to each other and our relationship. Yet, much as we discussed the possibility of moving in together, we never seriously planned to create our own household. Part of it was the fear that our eternal courtship would evaporate in the process; part was the objective difficulty of getting me professionally set up in San Diego, an area saturated with PhDs at a time when retiring full-time professors were being replaced by adjuncts. But part of it was also our commitment to our respective children, and the fear that our partnership would threaten their financial future in some way.

In the summer of 1996 Sara finally came to visit me again. Her friend Laura was with her this time as well. They had finished high school and were a bit more mature. We went to a café and over a cappuccino I looked at them and said, "I have two really nice-looking young women, and I haven't had to do much to get them either. Isn't that nice?"

"Right, it's nice for you," Laura said. Her parents were also separated, and she lived with her mother. "My father provides for me. In Italy, a parent has that obligation until a child is twenty-five years old."

Sara said nothing, but her eyes egged her friend on.

"Why do you bring this up?" I asked.

"Because you too have obligations, but aren't heeding them," Sara answered. "Dad supports me and you don't contribute."

"Do you mean that you need my help to go to college?" I asked.

"Maybe," she answered.

"Well, I didn't know you wanted to go to college, but if that's the case, I'll do what I can."

Sara asked me about my mother, Delia: Who was she? How did she die? What is memorable about her? It made me cry. I realized she had never known about me except through what others said. This curiosity made me feel like she needed me—perhaps the time had come for her to come toward me. I told her about Delia—the way she raised me to be equal, how I had found it difficult to live up to that back home.

"People think I'm no good because you live so far away," she observed.

"They think the same of me because you live so far away. Perhaps we can become friends and people will respect us more. What do you think?" I asked.

"Why are you no longer teaching?" she asked. "Why are you no longer studying?" I replied.

I told her the story of my family and we decided I'd go back to teaching and support her.

Part Two:
Origins

Dear Sara,
I know I haven't been the most desirable parent, but please listen to the story of your mother's family and the circumstances, desires, and illusions which brought her to the so-called new world.

XIV
An Unconventional Family

Your grandmother died of cancer in 1968. It was the first time that I was seriously hurt by the failure of modern medicine. My parents were leftist intellectuals in Rome, where Grandma taught *lettere,* including Italian, history, geography, and Latin. Delia was audacious and majestic, with her regal deportment and Titian-red hair. As a young woman, her style, beauty, and intelligence had been enough to intimidate any man. She had been raised in Rome by Neapolitan parents who, due to the unification of Italy, had moved to the capital of the new state. Her father, Gaspare, was a judge; her mother, Angela, a seamstress, a job she quit to get married. As the family story went, Angela's natural beauty had earned the attention of a higher-class suitor, and Gaspare had managed to charm her in turn with his forensic eloquence. Their two daughters, Delia and Irene, had received first-class educations, partly because there were no sons to compete for the resources of the family. When Grandpa Dario met Delia, she was a cultured, brilliant, and elegant *Laureata in lettere* assigned to teach in the school district of Veltri, a provincial town northeast of Rome where he lived with his family. She had chosen Montessorian education as her philosophy and field of experimental research. From her perspective, your grandpa Dario was but a *giovane di belle speranze,* a young guy with good hopes and little else to his credit. He looked inspired, serious, and intense, with his translucent skin and mobile gaze. She agreed to marry him on condition that, eventually, they establish their residence in Rome, the "eternal city," or *urbs,* as the Romans called it.

My paternal grandmother Teresa died when you were three years old. Her first-born, Dario, was a self-proclaimed atheist who, in 1952, agreed to marry in the church so as to not completely shock his own parents and Delia's. Yet Teresa cried throughout the service, for the condition was that Dario and Delia's marriage be classified as one of mixed religions, with hers being "Catholic" and his "Atheist." It was a union of opposites. Delia was to Dario like the ocean to the mountain, the sun to the moon, the city to the country, the socialite to the peasant. The combination was not devoid of management problems, which, as their firstborn, I was privileged to watch from a seat in the first row.

When they returned to the capital, Delia's enthusiasm for Montessori education made her part of the pedagogical avant-garde of the nation, as she was invited to participate in a pilot program that applied the Montessori method to the middle-school system.

Having paid their duties to Italian family traditions and Catholicism, Delia and Dario proceeded to worship literature, art, and politics, the three lay religions of my home. Not a single copy of the Bible was allowed on our overflowing bookshelves, for, as they explained, the "book of books," in both its parts of the Old and the New Testament, made claims to being the only book necessary, and this very idea would deter young minds from desiring new knowledge.

Your uncle Andrea was born in 1958, the year your grandpa was first elected as a congressman, at which point, for all practical purposes, he turned his paternal authority over to Delia. At the time Italy had no divorce laws, but she could have gotten rid of him any time through the Vatican annulment process, had she simply and even falsely claimed that he prevented her from giving your uncle Andrea and I a Catholic education. And precisely because she did not care to raise us in any religious faith, the situation put her positively in charge of the family.

With her knowledge of many languages, her familiarity with Marxism, her deep faith in Montessorianism, your grandma banned the fears and repressions traditionally associated with Catholicism from the environment for us to grow. She raised Andrea and I as absolute equals, and that included buying unisex clothes that could be passed from girl to boy. I fantasized about ruffled pink dresses with frills and bows like every other little girl.

"It's so pretty!" I'd exclaim as we passed shop windows that had them on display.

Grandma Delia would keep going. "That stuff has no style at all," she'd comment as she pulled my hand. Andrea looked puzzled at his sweaters that buttoned on the left. Delia explained, "It was your sister Gaia's. We can afford much higher quality this way."

She also banned toys that induced gender-specific behavior. "I don't want you to play with dolls, Gaia," she explained, "and I don't want you, Andrea, to play with weapons." The ban was extended to all members of the family, with grannies and other relatives planning their gifts accordingly. Our creative talents were encouraged. I liked drawing and painting, and so pencils, watercolors, and gouache became my domains. Andrea was more construction oriented. He enjoyed Legos and model railroads and trains, and had a musical talent that earned him music lessons. We liked each other and were friends rather than competitors. We were trusted and trusting in turn, which made us happy, the trust of our parents being well worth the few boundaries they set.

In 1961, when the first Italian public television channel began broadcasting, your grandma was invited to teach history in the instructional programs designed to widen the country's cultural literacy base. It was her second job, and a promise for a new career. At that point, TV sets were not common, and Andrea and I used to watch her at Signora Augusta's, a neighbor whose apartment was opposite to us on the second floor. The TV set was in the kitchen, and several neighbors joined to watch. Only Delia's bust was visible, which puzzled your uncle Andrea.

"Is *Mamma* going to come home all in one piece?"

Signora Augusta explained, "She's not really inside this TV set, dear. It's an image that everyone can see if they have one."

"So her legs are still on?"

"Trust me, Andrea, your *mamma* is safe. There's no reason to worry."

Your grandma's TV class was a success, and the following year they asked her again.

"Should I continue or give it up?" she asked me, as Andrea played in her lap. Your grandfather's career in politics was taking off, and she did not have enough of his support at home. Eventually, she decided to spend more time with us, gave up her pilot program and moved to a conventional school closer to home. As the 1960s came into full sway, she was being fairly successful in reconciling her responsibilities, but something about her dreams had been lost.

One could well claim that your grandma was a casualty of Grandpa's career in politics, even though, ironically, Dario might have felt his choice of such a demanding career was a result of his marriage to the daughter of a highly positioned professional. Delia saw herself as an equal to her husband. Early on in their relationship, she had established herself as his primary interlocutor, like the philosophers Simone De Beauvoir and Jean-Paul Sartre. But I think that when he became a politician she felt betrayed, not so much because of the admirers that came with his success, but because he no longer trusted her as a friend. His public image became more important, and this required a wife who'd agree with him on everything—one with scarcely any ideas of her own. Motherhood enhanced her sense of embodiment, and, in the misogynist mentality of those times, this amounted to having one's brains flushed down one's fallopian tubes. So, as a politician's wife, Grandma found out that when push comes to shove men's true interlocutors are other men. Besides, Dario was picky and not willing to do what it took to be successful at his job. As you probably knew, the party in power since 1948 was a centrist political organization called Democrazia Cristiana, or Christian Democracy, largely controlled by the Catholic Church. In 1963 it decided to have the smaller Socialist Party join it in the country's administration. Grandpa was called to be a vice minister in the new cabinet, at the Treasury, and he accepted. A while later, the cabinet was reshuffled—which was very common—and he was invited to join again.

He told Delia about his misgivings at the dinner table. "The atmosphere of corruption and incompetence is overwhelming," he said. "I want to go back to being a simple congressman."

"That's a bit too heroic," Grandma cautioned. "Be sure to know what you're doing."

"What is right for the country is right for me," Dario declared. "Honey, I'm sure you understand."

Grandma said nothing, but I think she reflected on how his honesty would affect the family. She felt the decision had not been really made together.

The first signs of a potential health problem came from an accident that happened at home. While storing some preserves up high in the kitchen cabinets, Grandma fell from a ladder and broke her upper arm. For several weeks she was in a cast all the way down to her waist. Her beautiful breasts that had never known a bra felt trapped and breathless. This crisis gave her time to reflect.

"Who am I now? What have my dreams turned into? Is my husband still in love with me?" she thought.

In the mid-1960s the Italian feminist movement was waiting to happen. Career opportunities were much better for men; women did all the housekeeping and parenting; and there was no divorce. As a result, many Italian men practiced nonmonogamy, of the one-way sort. A few years into their marriage, they'd find someone else, and, in the best of cases, pretended they hadn't and carried on. Grandma's father, your great-grandpa Gaspare, was one of them. Their wives were often aware of what was going on, and put up with the situation for the sake of peace in the family. These women were known as *le cornute,* the cuckolded females. Supposedly, their juices would dry out, and they would inevitably flounder between obsessive hygiene and hysterical behavior. They swallowed their pride for fear that he would definitely choose *her*. But in her early years as a paid professional, Grandma Delia had fought for her own mother's dignity. She had helped your great-grandma Angela get a legal separation with a reasonable alimony. In empowering her own mother to free herself of a husband who no longer deserved her, Delia acted like a protofeminist. Angela now had her own place and did no free work for no man. She enjoyed her afternoons at a nearby café, a veil of lipstick on, hair rolled up, the beautiful white of her teeth on display. A cup of gelato was on the table in the wide sidewalk terrace. The chocolate bites melted between Angela's tongue and palate. If old admirers had still been around, I bet they would have been delighted to watch. I remember I was. Angela no longer was a *cornuta,* but a woman with her own dignity and happiness.

"I have done this for her," Delia thought. "My husband knows I would do the same for myself. If there is someone else, wouldn't he tell me? Wouldn't he have the decency to let me take control of my life again?"

With her breasts wrapped in her cast, Grandma Delia must have pondered these questions. Perhaps she was still waiting for a move from him.

"Doesn't he owe me the debt of honesty?" she might have asked herself.

This doubt, I bet, caused her mind to intercept the work of the healing system and her bloodstream failed to flush out the first newly formed cancer cells. The early clusters of her tumor were formed.

XV
Delia

ROME, THE 1960s

Before I married your father I had lived in two places with my family. The first apartment was sunny and spacious, with wide windows overlooking the fields teeming with new buildings or *palazzine* in a new development near the Vatican. The dust of construction sites subsided as the fields were conquered by urban sprawl. The buildings had three or four stories, with roll-up windows and stores on the ground floor. Our apartment was on the third floor. The drawing room had a warm wooden floor, and your grandma Delia made it into the children's room, our special space to experiment and grow. An old-fashioned lifestyle still prevailed in the neighborhood. A blue neon sign on the first floor said *latteria,* for the old-style dairy convenience store. Lea, the *portiera,* had a gentle smile and wavy brown hair cropped at the nape of her neck. She used to babysit for us in the porter's lodge, where I would read Pinocchio stories to her little girl. St. Peter's, with its procession of pilgrims and crowds of faithful, emanated a powerful aura of sacred energy. Strong wafts of incense brought waves of spiritual energy to our humble atheist abode. I missed that smell when we moved on, in 1964; I was eight and had no idea what it was.

From that apartment, your grandma sent me to the only public grade school that used the Montessori method, on the other side of town. Villa Paganini, in the Nomentana area, was a public park with Mediterranean pines and gravel. The school was in its heart, a series of well-aired and spacious wooden pavilions of a light-green color. The light entered our classroom windows with the rustle of tree branches. The small tables and independent chairs were arranged in irregular patterns, some for students who worked alone, some for groups of three or four. The learning materials we could choose from were stored in low shelves at the center and corners. They had natural textures and colors that felt magically alive as we observed them and held them in our hands. Some activities required blindfolding which activated one's sense of touch or smell. We trusted our surroundings completely, with the teacher as the loving force behind this joy. Our beautiful creations and projects decorated the walls.

In post–World War II Italy, the impulse to renew the system was as strong as the guilt of a nation that had failed to stop the raise of Fascism. Your grandparents went to school while Fascism loomed large on the cultural landscape, and wanted their children's experience of education to be completely different from theirs. Montessori's method rejected authority for inner motivation, a collaborative spirit, and a sense of reverence for knowledge. That's how I learned how to learn and to love learning, and could not know how fortunate I was. Like your grandma, and Montessori herself, I still believe that education is the most effective way to multiply the joy and peace of the world.

As I entered fourth grade, we moved to Monte Mario, a more prestigious neighborhood on a hill a few minutes away from our first home. Delia's father had moved there since the separation, and bought the apartment next to his own for his daughter's family. Your great-aunt Irene refused, and so the offer came to your grandma Delia. Grandpa Dario encouraged her to accept.

"It's going to work out for us," he said as he stood near the desk.

"I'm not sure I want to live near my dad," Delia replied, "besides, the place is claustrophobic. Don't you think we can do better on our own?"

"I'd take it, dear," Dario said. "You never know."

The apartment was bigger and the area more upscale. But the place was dark, noisy, and disconnected from the territory. The large highrise building stood on a steep slope, its greenish yellow brick and plaster façade studded with diminutive half-moon balconies on which nothing would grow because they overlooked a major traffic road. The city bus that stopped at the corner offered twenty-four-hour service. A gray, tubular courtyard was at the center of the building, lined with kitchen windows looking into each other. Ours was at the bottom where the sunlight never reached it directly. Remember how dark that kitchen still was when you lived there with your dad? Grandma Delia had had the place remodeled, with a walk-in closet in the master bedroom, large closets, cabinets and shelves wherever possible, and a wall-to-wall mirror in the main bathroom. The decorations were classy and extravagant. The large drawing room, in a classical style, was for entertaining, with wide flowing curtains and fine porcelain. The study, more modern, was for the family, its two main walls covered with top-down bookshelves. Paintings by contemporary artists decorated the walls. The nude was a major theme, with inked-in drawings of male and female bodies in natural poses. Delia managed to ooze some of her solar style on to the place—even though by the time you and your dad moved in it had been lost. Still, as you remember, turning the lights on for cooking was always necessary, and the screeching sound of the bus brakes punctuated our sleep all night long.

Yet the artificial glow of the place did not quite manage to compensate for its basic structural problems, and I felt the values it inspired were also unhealthy. It encouraged obsession and mental constipation. When I was a child, meat was a prestige food and its proteins were considered irreplaceable, while vegetable proteins were considered premodern—the diet of peasants. But I must have been an innate vegetarian for I hated red meat and could barely swallow it. I remember myself way past lunchtime at the kitchen table, the neon light already turned on, a gray wall behind the pane, mother watching me eat the last bit of meat on my plate.

"Can I leave this, *Mamma?*" I'd ask.

"You know you can't. Meat has proteins and you need them to grow well."

"I can't swallow it," I'd reply, my eyeballs nearly out of their sockets, as the chewed food made me gag.

"It's only a matter of will, dear. Now, keep going."

As mother turned around, I'd spit the mush into my palm and throw it under the seat. I suspected she was aware of my surreptitious behavior but never said a thing.

Your grandmother Delia wanted your uncle Andrea and I to be fluent in French, the international language which had freed some thinking space for Italian dissenters when she was young, in the Fascist era. Bilingualism was part of her program to build democracy through education. The bigger apartment meant we could afford some help, so she hired French au pairs. Martine was witty and energetic and her Parisian looks made a splash in our family. Her duties included using only French with Andrea and myself. We responded well and French became an intimate language we used in our games.

"Je dois aller aux toilettes," Andrea would say. I have to go to the bathroom.

"D'accord," Martine would reply. Okay.

"Peux-tu m'accompagner?" Can you take me?

"Mais non, tu es grand, voyons, tu peux faire tout seul." Come on, big boy, you can manage by yourself.

Martine had the prettiest French nose, and puffy lips in a heart shape. She had the most charming manners and wore black ballerina shoes and a white ribbon in her hair. When we went on vacation in the Alps, as was customary, your great-grandpa Gaspare promptly proceeded to make advances to her.

"Shame on you!" said Delia as Gaspare walked with his cane.

"I didn't do anything," he objected. "I just told her how charming she was!" his silky hands on the cane's ivory handle.

"What makes you think she'd be interested?" Delia retorted. *She's got enough men her age to keep at bay,* Grandma Delia must have thought as she decided to look for less exotic help.

With our bilingualism established, mother opted for Italian au pairs. In towns too far away from a university for a daily commute, many young women were ready to get a university education provided they found a part-time job cum place to stay. Delia's au pairs got room and board in Rome, some pocket money, time to themselves, and the support of a woman who already had the *Laurea* they sought. Marisa, from Positano—an enchanting beach town on the Gulf of Naples—was petite and extroverted in a truly Neapolitan way. Dina was from Todi, a medieval town in the Orvieto province, where Grandpa Dario was elected. Sensitive and self-possessed, she worked hard in an unpretentious way. Your grandma was sisterly, maternal, and protective in her customary protofeminist way. She cared that the au pairs meet their goals and complete their program, and was on their side as they struggled through, all the while knowing that when they succeeded she would have to replace them. They prolonged their stay, Marisa, from the agreed-upon three months to three years, Dina until after your grandma's premature death and her own *Laurea,* at which time she married a relative from grandpa's side of the family. To complete the household staff, Delia also hired Clara, a part-time cleaning lady. She was a single mother who had managed to gain respect for herself and her daughter with her hard work. Clara's Northern manners made her quite resourceful and independent. These women became part of our family, accepting the rules mother created, and providing Delia with a longed-for female companionship at home.

Delia had learned to love her body from the classics. She wanted this love to be the norm for her children, something they would not have to conquer again. She had absorbed the values of beauty and harmony of that older world, and, like a neo-pagan, she raised Andrea and me on Greek mythology, Sappho, and Ovid. The single and free Diana, goddess of wild nature, protector of women, became my favorite deity.

Mother created a clothing-optional home where one was free to be dressed, but covering oneself was not mandatory. No body part was shameful, no function too intimate to share. Clothes were embellishments necessary for receiving guests, going out, and staying warm, but within the family walls, the body in all its parts was freely displayed. There were no locks on bathroom doors, and Andrea and I bathed together, with the au pairs supervising the ablutions.

"Stop splashing me, Gaia!" Andrea would say. I'd keep going.

"Can't you leave him alone?" Dina asked.

"All right, all right, I will," I replied as I continued to play.

That's how you found out boys had penises and never envied them, for "your reproductive organs are inside, in your belly," as mother explained when the ablutions came to an end, "and they are a lot more complex and necessary."

In the wall-to-wall mirror that decorated the large bathroom, Delia's generous body was often on display. Her skin was smooth with gold tones that tanned to sienna. Her shape a mixture of Juno's and Venus's, as the Romans would say. A fresh torso on top of a high waist sported a round pair of shoulders and toned-up breasts. A turned-up navel on top a gently curved belly lead to her portly hips and thighs, and the abundant pubic curls.

"When am I going to get pubic hair?" I asked one day, looking up at her majestic shape.

"When your puberty starts, dear. Your breasts will bud and you'll flesh up," she replied touching my skinny shoulder blades.

Dario would rarely participate in our bathroom conversations. He was both less proud of his body and more shameful. His legs were thin and crooked, his shoulders stooped, his skin too pale. Yet he was sexy in his own disarming way.

It was a great way to be a family, but the rest of the world was not that far ahead. Occasional clashes with adjoining institutions happened, as with my art teacher in eighth grade. Public middle schools were generally coed, with boys and girls in separate classrooms exchanging furtive glances in the hallways. A classroom's walls were usually bare, except for a Crucifix and a portrait of the president, the twin icons under which Italian public education is still dispensed. On the floor below the icons was a pedestal on which stood the high teacher's desk, or cathedra. I was good at drawing and I was often among my art teachers' favorite students. In eighth grade my art teacher was an elderly lady with white hair who had never been married. At free drawing practice, Miss Fortini would just tell us girls to draw a subject of our choice. I had noticed the china ink drawing in the study at home, a ripe female body with generous hips and wavy hair, sitting on her bed. *It looks like Delia,* I thought. The next day I went up to the teacher's desk and presented a nude drawing of my *mamma,* seated and slightly turned toward a plate held in her right hand. That year Delia was a teacher at my school also. The drawing portrayed a full-bodied female figure, neither exceedingly "feminine" nor exceedingly "maternal."

"Who's this woman?" Miss Fortini asked, embarrassed.

"My mom!" I replied, glancing at her.

"Perhaps it's best for you to take this drawing back home, then."

"Okay," I said, vexed.

"Can you please do this assignment again?" Miss Fortini asked. I nodded and went back to my desk.

"What could be wrong with this drawing?" Delia asked at the dining table.

"Delia, you know how petty teachers can be," Dario said.

"It's a fine drawing," she insisted.

"That's what I thought," I said.

I came up with a new version of my mom's body and gave it to the teacher again. Miss Fortini was even more embarrassed but still afraid to tell me that this was shameful, that it was pornography, and that I had to change the subject altogether.

"I'm afraid this won't do either," she commented.

Perhaps the teacher was aware of Delia's ideas—afraid to confront her. The room was silent and on edge. Buried behind their desks, the girls observed. They knew about keeping one's legs closed. Their attire marked their progress toward fertile womanhood; silk stockings and garter belts if you had your period, knee-high white cotton socks if you were still waiting. They were giddy and restless.

Oblivious to the general embarrassment, I wanted the principles of my home to apply in school as well. When I was on the third version, Miss Fortini realized I was not going to clothe my nude, and tore up my drawing altogether.

"I have to do a different drawing," I told Delia at dinner.

"We'll talk to Dad about art lessons," she replied.

"Art lessons with a real painter and live models?" I asked, excited.

"Why not?" Delia said. "Isn't that what you wanted?"

"Of course!" I replied.

She arranged for weekly lessons with an older female painter whose study was filled with exciting smells and well-formed female models whose tawny skins and purple nipples were on display. There my passion for the nude and for the female body developed, and I will always be grateful to my mother for the gift of loving female bodies I first learned from her.

Your grandma's premature, tragic death attached ugly images of decay to my memory. When her cast was removed, she did a lot of physiotherapy, followed by an incubation period. She felt constipated. "It must be hemorrhoids," the doctor said while her life went on as before. She was beautiful and admired, successful and independent, yet something didn't work, and she failed to make the necessary changes in a timely way.

Her colon cancer was diagnosed at an advanced stage, but surgery was still possible. The surgeon removed her colon and most of her lower intestines, and replaced her anus with an artificial opening on her abdomen. But the sphincter could not be replaced, which is why at all times Grandma wore a pouch on top of her artificial anus on her belly. There were no support programs for recovering patients, and their will was considered irrelevant to their healing process. Surgeons did not inform them they were about to die and told their spouses instead.

I am not sure that mother would have been happy to live to an elderly age, now that her body wasn't much to be proud of. The first months were difficult, looking for clothes that would hang loose and stand off her belly, making sure that the pouch was always clean and properly placed, telling people about her new condition so they would not be surprised if something went off. But with her customary pride, your grandma did well. She might have believed what the doctors told her, that the tumor was benign and would not come back. Grandpa Dario got closer to her, admiring her courage. But then, there was no stopping the cancer's progress, for Grandma's will had not been activated, and the same belief system surrounded her. And soon it was radiation and chemotherapy.

The disintegration process was relentless. It encroached upon the popular belief that modern scientific progress can defeat illness and pain. I remember Mother's statuary body stooped down by radiation and shriveled by chemotherapy, as she dragged her feet from room to room in a flannel robe, her hair now white in disheveled waves, her diaphanous face pale with death. She had still not been told what she had, as was customary.

In her agony, silence was the most unbearable pain. Silence about what was intuitively evident, and yet unspoken in the gaping *omertà* of all involved. It was the last year in which Andrea and I had a mother at all. If at least she could have yelled, "I'm dying. Has anybody noticed?" If we could have at least spent it cuddling her, comforting her, telling her how lovely she was, and how grateful we were for all her wonderful gifts. But we had no permission to do that. The appearance of normalcy had to be kept up at all times. Grandma had to pretend she believed she was going to get well, and we had to pretend we believed her pretense. Demonstrating any kind of special affection could have compromised this façade and was therefore considered dangerous rather than merciful. Grandpa Dario dealt with the problem by being around as little as possible; we and other relatives followed suit. Acting our part was too difficult, so we would rather not play. A small measure of compassion came from the household help. Perhaps less emotionally involved, Dina and Clara were able to negotiate an easier role to play.

Because he believed there was no hope, as the doctor said, Dario avoided her and spent time at Marina's, his former girlfriend who had married a GI at the end of the war. But Delia's female friends from her student days often came to cheer her up, and once she was on the phone with one of them.

"This illness will not forgive me," she said. "It won't let me off."

I scribbled the words down on a piece of paper, as I often did carelessly. But this time my doodles were dangerous. When Delia saw the paper, she took it with her and asked questions of Dario as he came home.

"What does this mean? Does Gaia know anything you haven't told me? Talk to me!"

He replied, calmly, "There's nothing to know, my dear. You've got nothing serious—trust me. You'll be well in no time at all."

The questions stopped. Dario was relieved, and I learned never to carelessly doodle again.

Why me? Delia must have thought as her body declined further, *I never whined, never smoked, never drank . . .Why?* Inevitably, her illness felt like a punishment for not being a more deferential wife to my dad.

I grew more distant, wondering, *What if more questions came? How many denials, how many silences can I sustain?* I kept going out with my friends and became aware that I was going to lose her only two weeks ahead of time. I never did say good-bye in a loving way. But I remember my guilty sense of joy when I found out she was being sent to a private clinic again. "It's the best place for her to die," Dario and the doctors agreed in their secret talks.

Miniskirts were the latest rage, and Delia felt that girls who wore them could lose their centeredness from overexposure to the male gaze. The new rage allowed me to show my legs in full length and the excitement assuaged my pain. When Delia had been gone for a few days, I went to an after school party in one of my favorite miniskirts. The guy I hoped to meet did not show. I got depressed and went home early. Dina was cooking dinner, extending her services beyond the call of duty.

She looked at my exposed legs. "Is something wrong?" she said.

"Well, Dina, people keep telling me that *Mamma* is going to get better, but I only see her getting worse."

Dina turned her face to the stove again without a word. "Get yourself ready for dinner," she said after a moment.

In the materialistic culture of modernity, my teenager's life was full of conflicting emotions, as my mother was dying and no one was supposed to know. Eroticism, my only access to the sacred, helped to soften the acrid smell of death.

I last saw my mother alive in a hospital bed. Grandpa Dario almost forced me to visit her, for he knew she was close to the end. I showed up sporting my long legs in a vertiginous miniskirt. She made no comment.

"How is school?" she asked.

She was pale, her skin almost transparent. Her mother, Angela, glanced at me as if to alert me to something indecorous.

Mother looked at both of us and said, "I feel urine pulsating in my blood, up to my fingertips," to which she pointed.

In late February 1968, bare trees filled the white air and the room smelled of medications. On March 7 we went to your grandma's funeral. Delia had died of renal block, her kidneys dissolving into an amoebic mass of cancer cells. One of the most beautiful, elegant, and intelligent women in her social circle—her husband's political career the object of people's envy—was gone. Great-grandfather Gaspare bent on the open casket and touched her bloodless hands.

"Forgive me, Delia. My turn should've come first," he said and kissed her forehead. We moved into the procession and on to the cemetery. As I surreptitiously raised my head to glance at the people behind the hearse, I realized I was now being looked upon as an "orphan," a child marked for trouble and no longer to be envied.

As my life went on, the memory of a healthy mother gradually replaced the images of decay. I remember my mother vividly, and the sumptuous, solar beauty of her body still dazzles me. Perhaps Delia liked to show it off, and it was pushy of her to expect nudist behavior from all members in the family. But it is an assertiveness I love for it helped me access a joyful sense of my embodied self. In my living room, I still have the drawing that inspired the nudes I did of your grandma. When I hear stories of young girls whose lost mothers live in their memory as a body of love—a body of eros—the narrative touches me as a structure of feeling I can call my own.

XVI
Winds of Change

It was the momentous year of 1968, with its uprisings and widespread movements for social change. Observers might have dubbed the "eternal city" as one "too old" to play a major role in its making. Yes, we know that Rome, or *urbs,* "the city," as the Romans call it, is still somewhat peripheral with respect to the European context. But it turned out to be a major player in the actualization of the changes that were to make those years famous.

Precisely because most Romans lived near the headquarters of Catholicism, they knew enough about that religion to have it be more than a set of formalities. In those times, very few people had any authentic religious faith, including your maternal grandparents. Catholicism had caused several disappointments. In the nineteenth century, the Papal States occupied the best part of central Italy and divided the industrialized North from the rural South, or *Meridione.* Their presence had considerably delayed the country's process of modernization, which is why patriotism was tinged with anticlericalism. Ever since the unification, in 1870, the papacy considered itself a prisoner of the Italian State. Eventually, in 1929, about halfway through his Fascist *ventennio,* Mussolini brokered a truce with the church government, trading papal acceptance for the Italian State against the status of state religion for Catholicism. Later on, Pope Pious XII became famous for failing to take a stand against the Holocaust. When your grandparents arrived, the pope and his Vatican center of operations were considered a social-control system and a big show. While my grandparents had been raised in God's fear, your grandma Delia was an agnostic, Grandfather Dario an atheist. As literature majors, they had intellectual aspirations, and elected art, literature, and politics as the three religions of our home. Both were schoolteachers and Grandpa became a politician later on.

In the sixteenth year of her marriage, mother had been the main source of authority in our family, and she was dying, while in Europe a major sexual revolution was getting into full sway. I will never know in what ways her life would have been transformed had she lived on. Your grandma was an assertive person with high expectations of me, her daughter. While she was alive the world never felt like a sexist or violent place, even though sometimes I felt she was, for nothing but perfection would satisfy her. And with her absolute faith in my ability to learn anything, she'd obtain quite a lot. As a classicist, she wanted me to get an early start in the wisdom of the ancients and used the summer after my elementary school graduation for that purpose. I remember spending my vacation learning Latin declensions for her. We were in the Alps, and my nostrils tingled with the scent of pine trees around the garden table where we worked.

I delivered as usual. As I entered junior high, I enrolled in the school where she taught. Your grandma was proud to have me there, and used to explain that I had to grow up strong *because* I was a girl. As an adult, I would have to be a go-getter, for professional opportunities would not fall in my lap as happened to mediocre men. One time she went as far as telling on me to my teacher, for she knew I had skipped my homework.

"Call her on it," she recommended.

"But I've got lots to do. I'm behind with my program," her colleague said.

"Set an example for the whole group," Mother urged.

Black smocks and white collars were the school uniform. There were about thirty of us girls in the classroom.

"Cosentini," the teacher said. "Have you done your homework?"

I blushed and lowered my gaze. Then I stood up as was customary when a teacher called you. The girls watched me as my negligence was confessed in this public way. Of course, it all was very confusing then, but those lessons made a lot of sense later on.

Il sessantotto was approaching—the momentous year of 1968, with student rebellions in Paris and revolutionary winds blowing over to us from nearby France. Your grandma passed away on March 5, and I will never know how she would have responded to the new era. In that experimental age I was left to raise myself, and became sexually active at an early age. I was only fourteen, but I had to have a boyfriend. You might find this weird, but believe me, it made me feel closer to a body, compensating for the loss of my mother's body. I loved demure, feminine boys who wouldn't presume to take the initiative and responded on cue to my jagged intimations. We went quite far, but not "all the way." I remember my first French kiss in the garden of a girlfriend's house in the Alps, near Geneva, where we were on vacation. Smell of trees and fresh skin dry from the mountain air, a thin body and blond, straight hair; sweet lips together; moist tongues touching as we shush each other's hair.

Then there was Roberto, a schoolmate with a motorcycle both of us used to ride back home. I held on to my backseat as he drove, sporting my thighs in a miniskirt. In the street, at bus stops, men stood with eyes wide open as we passed provocatively in a wave of erotic energy. We often ended up at his place and spent time in bed; a lavender spread on the twin bed; a door ajar; us lying down in our clothes; distant clatter from the kitchen stove; the Mamas and the Papas on the stereo; *The Graduate;* sometimes it was Mick Jagger in "Let's Spend the Night Together." Under his fly the soft bulge of an erection.

"Put your hands down there!"

"Like this?"

"No, inside."

Mushy flesh. Pulsating veins. Hands nudging around my genitals.

"What's happening to my panties?"

My labia became soft with wetness. That breathing of body against body, that pressure of crotch against crotch under our clothes, the intrusion of innocent hands in our genital areas were exploring and adventurous, making me very warm with excitement and sometimes I'd feel a soft sense of fulfillment and elation. This behavior felt perfectly normal, but when your grandfather Dario discovered it he sent me to a Florence convent.

In the wake of the revolution of 1968, militants in the student movement were experimenting with eroticizing public and institutional spaces. Making love in a park or an occupied university was considered brave. It was regarded as a playful and effective way to surprise authorities and their system of law enforcement. For many women my age, this particular defiance of law and order meant emancipation from the sex-gender system that placed our highest value between our legs. We had been raised to believe that, as women, we were the repositories of emotions and were capable of little else. Men, on the other hand, had been trained to separate feelings from sex. Some of them did it systematically and quite successfully. They had feelings for a wife, to whom they were affectionate, *"Sai io a mia moglie voglio tanto bene"*—You know, I'm so very fond of my wife. Passion and good sex for a mistress: *"Con lei ci faccio le cose zozze, mi sfogo"*—With her it gets really dirty. I feel liberated. Obviously, both wives and mistresses were considered too sentimental to sustain similar arrangements for themselves.

As aspiring feminists of that famous second-wave generation, we wanted to demonstrate that sentimentality was neither our nature nor our destiny. This was an important statement for it was a way to proclaim that we, too, were capable of separating emotional involvement from sexual pleasure. We were eagerly intent in demonstrating, primarily to ourselves, that women's monogamy is not more natural than men's. It simply was a cultural construct designed to control female sexual expression based on the system of retaliation that gave a bad reputation to "promiscuous" females. *Puttana*, slut, and *ragazza facile*, flirtatious girl, were the most common slurs. How come we women had to feel ashamed of the sexual prowess men were so proud of? What slurs would insult boys in the same way? I felt the sexual expression I experienced at that young age was part of a larger experiment in envisaging the world our generation wanted to reinvent. Of course, we did not manage to correct all the mistakes, but in our mind sexual experiments were not even remotely connected with abuse or shame, and they were ever so more emotionally intense as they involved the exploration of our respective young bodies and their different erotic mechanisms.

As you might expect, Grandpa did not feel the same way. He was born in the heart of the Apennines, the stalwart mountain chain that forms the Italian peninsula's backbone in Fosca, a town of subsistence farmers and shepherds. The timbered mountain slope came down to a narrow valley where the river flew, icy and transparent. Two main roads intersected on the valley floor. And that's where Grandpa's parents met and raised their family, in a historic building dated from the eighteenth century. Antonio, your great-grandfather, arrived in Fosca in 1912. He was a *maestro,* a schoolteacher sent by the central government to provide basic instruction to the children of the mostly illiterate local peasants. He taught all of them in a one-room school, juggling between the multiple levels. Just like other supporters of the country's unification, he had faith in Catholicism but was suspicious of the clergy. He was law-abiding and *pacioccone,* a happy-go-lucky type of fellow whose chubby face inspired peace and common sense.

In Fosca he met your great-grandmother Teresa. She was the eldest daughter of the local pharmacist, whose family had been part of the minuscule and impoverished local aristocracy. There, educating girls beyond the elementary level was not customary, since a family's paltry resources would be better invested in a son's preparation for a professional career reserved for men, such as the law or medicine. Great-grandma Teresa had been raised to get up at 4 a.m. and bake with the maids. She knew all the chores in the home-based production system upon which the town's rural economy was based. Her specialty was making capons, which was done by opening a cockerel's abdomen and wrapping a rope around its balls tight enough that they'd eventually fall off. She traded this skill against other favors in the local barter system. When her only brother, Dario, died in World War I the opportunity for a daughter's education arose, but she had been several years out of school already and so her younger sister was chosen. Grandpa Dario was Teresa's firstborn, followed by another boy. He was named after his late uncle, a *caduto per la patria,* one who fell for his homeland and surely deserved this honor. Dario was Teresa's favorite child, considered a prodigy due to his diligence and intelligence. Up to the equivalent of ninth or tenth grade, both sons were tutored by their own father Antonio. They graduated as *privatisti,* or home-schooled students admitted to the state exams.

XVII
"Slut!"

As a widower, your grandfather was going back to his own ways. Having delegated authority to his wife now passed away, he was having problems keeping things under control. He had suffered his first stroke and was concerned about his health. But he did not go back to teaching, due to the better pay and his faith in politics. He was often away for work, which turned Dina into a frustrated all-time governess. Your grandfather's predicament was ironic for, as a socialist, he supported the 1968 *movimento,* but the movement's new erotic ethos summoned his ancestral fears and compelled him to exercise his patriarchal authority.

Abandoned by Delia, his public image at the mercy of the rebellious teen-ager your mother was, he seemed persuaded that preserving the value a female student holds between her legs was the essence of high school education.

True, girls were now being educated like boys, but what was the goal of that education if not turning girls into better mothers eventually? For Dario, a person's sexual activity started through initiation rather than trial and error. Young men were initiated by older women whose experience made them less than respectable, while "respectable" women were initiated by their husbands. Since Dario did not like my boyfriend Roberto, he thought I had been assaulted rather than consenting. Rape was called *violenza carnale,* a violation of the flesh, and the law considered it a crime against public decency, not its victims. There was no concept of marital rape, since a married woman accepted all of her husband's future advances when she said *"sì."* Public sex was not encouraged, but prosecutable assaults were those on virgins, since that was the seal that granted a woman's value as a marriage commodity. Indeed, up to a few generations earlier a rapist's "punishment" had been marrying his victim. This repaired the damage to the woman's family, while her will did not enter the equation at all.

A few months earlier, while driving through the Veltri valley, Dario had recommended celibacy to me. It was the first winter Mother was dead and a family friend had invited me for a skiing vacation.

I was sitting in the passenger seat when he said, "You should marry as a virgin." I kept looking straight ahead. "Your mother did," he added after a moment.

Why is he bringing this up at this time? I thought as I looked at him in dismay. "I never said I wouldn't," I replied.

I wondered if he realized he was talking about the body that hosted me in my prenatal state—a body whose hearse we had followed together to the cemetery. I thought of Delia's hymen once in the birth channel through which I had been born.

When Roberto and I started going steady, Grandpa Dario established a curfew schedule for me and started to beat me with his belt—one stroke for every minute I was late.

"It's eight-fifteen," he said one day when I came home.

I lay down on the couch on my belly and he undid his belt. I knew each whipping caused him pain for he must have known there was a better way.

When he was done, I got up and looked at his face. He was exhausted. I wondered what he'd do if I came home at 9 p.m.

Andrea and Dina waited for us at the kitchen table, but our appetite was gone. This seemed such a barbarian way to administer justice that I started to come home late on purpose, to dare him to execute his order.

When he decided not to let me go out at all, I invited Roberto at home. He was fun to play with, like one of those funky Cabbage Patch Kids you liked so much when you lived in California. I loved to help him with his homework. A bit short, a couple of bricks under his feet would have placed him slightly above my face, in the "right" position for him and I to play a kissing scene in Hollywood. I found out later his father had also recently passed away.

The hottest year in the Italian uprisings of the *movimento* was 1969. Emanuela was in my class and she was also having her first sexual experiments. Pretty in a defiant way, she had wide green eyes, high cheekbones, straight blonde hair, and a nice oval jaw. We two girls were part of the first generation of women raised to think that our minds were our most important assets. We didn't quite want to throw our virginity away, but didn't regard it as the certificate of warranty we'd later need to marry. We were involved in our first experiments as our girls' bodies were turning into women's bodies, and our boyfriends' into men's. According to the sexual ethos of the *movimento,* we shared our experiences in minutest detail. In the morning we met in the school bathroom to discuss our exploits while some boring class was going on.

"Lorenzo had an erection," Emanuela explained one day. "I could feel it pulsating under his pants."

"Yes, this happens to Roberto also," I replied. "It feels mushy and cozy to touch this swelling flesh."

"What a strange body part," Emanuela commented.

"It's fun to get to know it," I said.

"Aren't you happy that we can be sexual and still be considered respectable girls?" Emanuela asked.

"Yes," I replied, "but it would be nice to talk about these things with the boys as well."

Trying on the new freedom women in the *movimento* had made our friendship very strong, and in the afternoon at home we focused on our own bodies. The bathroom tile was a glowing yellow and an oval mirror over the lavatory reflected the beautiful budding breasts adorning our bare chests.

"Yours are especially attractive," I told Emanuela one day, "with their wide base and pointy nipples."

"Yours are prettier," Emanuela answered. "They're fuller and more curvy."

I stepped out and invited Andrea in for a verdict. He stood in the dark hallway while both of us were now turned toward the door.

"What do you think of our bosoms?" I asked. "Which one looks better?"

Poised at the doorframe, the boy looked thoughtful in his thin body and straight hair. "Both look fine to me," he said after a moment then went away.

In the mirror, Emanuela's face giggled as she looked at mine. I smiled and glared at our glowing chests. We could have turned to each other for sexual experiments. Did the thought cross our minds at all?

With Andrea growing up and Dina still at home, the study was temporarily turned into my bedroom. I started to read voraciously, passionate novels about adultery in the nineteenth century like *Madame Bovary* and *Anna Karenina*. I was grounded, and used to ask Roberto to visit me when everybody was already in bed—or so I thought. We'd lay on the sofa bed under the library, Emma and Anna surreptitiously watching our tryst from the bookshelves. He'd stay for about a half hour and we'd lie down chest against chest, feeling our bodies get turned on. But Dina became suspicious and got us trapped.

"Be careful as you cross the hallway," I said one night as he got ready to leave.

He kissed me good-bye. "I will," he said at the room's door.

I heard some noise near the entrance, then he was back.

"What's wrong?" I asked.

"The door's locked."

"Really?" I got up and crossed to the apartment's entrance. I turned the knob. The door was locked from the inside and I had no key. *Dina*, I thought. *She never locks from the inside, though.*

"I don't know," I whispered. "It could be an accident, but it could be intentional—to get you."

"What shall we do?" he asked, a bit scared.

"Well, you're locked in, so it's not our fault you're here. Why don't you stay? Dina opens early in the morning to get the trashcan back in."

He was slightly perplexed. "Okay," he said and came back toward the bedroom. Our bodies were kind of frozen, and we spent the night waiting for the light of day, a "first night" devoid of any charm or joy. At seven the entrance door was still locked.

Roberto was on edge. "What if somebody finds me in here?" he asked.

Andrea came in in his pajamas as he sometimes did on Sunday mornings. He looked at us.

"He was locked in," I explained.

Andrea made a worried face. "Why was the door locked?" he asked.

"I wish I knew," I said. "Can you help him to escape?"

"How?"

I got up and unmade the bed, then showed him the sheets twisted together in a rope. "The drawing room window looks onto the terrace below. You hold it and he climbs out from there."

Roberto looked perplexed. "You expect me to do that?"

"What else?" I said. "Do you want Dina to find you in here and get you arrested?"

They left together. A few minutes later Andrea was back.

"It went okay," he said and went back to his room.

This Romeo-and-Juliet type of escape avoided the flagrancy of having Dina find Roberto in my bed, but she still reported to Dario that I nightly received his visits in my bedroom.

Grandpa enlisted my high school principal to deal with me, and I offered minimal cooperation. The shabby office smelled of papers, with a gray light filtering through thin shutters. The principal, corpulent and balding, sat behind a large desk and looked at us through his thick lenses.

"Have a seat," he said.

"I need to transfer my daughter out," Grandpa said. "Discipline is not enforced well enough here, and I don't like what happens."

"We'll do the paperwork," the principal said. He supported the movement and knew me as a good student.

"Is there a problem?" he asked me.

"He may be overreacting," my impertinent face suggested as I shrugged my shoulders.

Grandpa looked at the principal, anxiously, then at me, enraged. *"Sgualdrina,"* he yelled, to save face and avoid the stronger *puttana* for whore. The insult still resonates within me in all its offensiveness. It occurred to me that there was no equivalent hate word for men. The principal kept his mouth shut, embarrassed. Grandpa signed the papers to transfer me out, and a few days later I moved to a Catholic boarding house in Florence. In the trauma of letting go of all my points of identity, it occurred to me as supremely ironic that to contain your mother's sense of adventure, your atheist grandfather would resort to a nuns' convent.

XVIII
Abuse

The boarding convent where Grandpa sent me next year was in Rome, in a modern *palazzina* in the west-end district of Monte Verde. At the nearby bus stop, the ivy-covered garden walls of the surrounding residential area intersected with the seedy inns of a nearby suburban ghetto, the Borgata del Trullo. A gated garden surrounded our building. The rooms were neat, with large windows and modern beds and desks. The hallway teemed with life, and a sense of community prevailed. We shared household chores and took buses to our respective public schools every day. The nuns cooked and supervised our work. Their light gray smocks tucked in at the waist did not quite hide their bodies curves, and their black caps left out the ends of their short hair. They were full of fun and zest, and did their work with a sense of humor.

In popular mythology, nuns were the butt of homophobic jokes, tribads who rubbed their bodies together. But at the evening prayer the convent's white, simple chapel vibrated with Gregorian chants, and one could sense our nuns' bodies alive and kicking under their gray habits. The absence of men encouraged trust and companionship between women, as in the romantic friendships of Ivy League women's colleges in the United States. My fellow boarder, Adriana, was sixteen, with red cheeks and tight lips, typical of the Sabine mountains near Veltri. Her father, a field worker, was dead, and her mother and sister struggled to survive on a meager pension. She was smart and perseverant, a bit guarded in consorting with the well-off. Her sturdy hips made me think of Fosca's peasants. I very chastely dated her, and every Sunday, with sister's permission, we went to the movies together. Another female friend, Clara, was pretty and not very daring. Our companionate lifestyle sublimated eroticism into good works. As the three of us visited the mentally ill and the bodily impaired, female spirituality provided a mode of access to the sacred that bypassed the male Christian god.

When I returned home, I continued to socialize with the differently abled. It was a way to deflect peer pressure by placing myself where gifts would not be thrown back in my face. On Sundays, with Adriana and Clara, I visited children and young patients in a mental institution in Rome, run by a religious order. Some visitors came from the boarding school for young victims of polio. It was there that I found my next boyfriend, to the utmost horror of my family. Lisandro was from Naples. His face, circled with black curls, opened up in a hearty smile like my grandmother Angela's. His body was rather athletic, but his left leg had been hit by polio, and was significantly weaker and shorter. With his special shoes, he had a firm step, but walked with a limp.

My family had changed so radically that I knew it was not a positive space for me to grow anymore. First, Grandpa Dario broke the friendship between Andrea and me, for I was "the bad example" he should not follow. Then Andrea became "more equal" and Dario enlisted his help to watch over me.

"You must not cover up for her," Grandpa explained to him. "Help me watch over her instead." Andrea looked up at him, puzzled. "Boys can have some fun," continued Dario, "but one has to control girls."

Then your grandfather called in *Nonna* Teresa, his widowed mom from Veltri, to do the housework. Teresa displayed a hardworking, no-nonsense, peasant type of behavior, but was no feminist. She dramatically changed our table rituals to reflect the patriarchal order. Grandpa ate steak because physicians believed it would keep his heart condition under control. We had regular two-course meals, pasta followed by meat and veggies. Needless to say, Grandpa's steak was just as expensive as our three meals put together. *Nonna* Teresa always served him first, with Andrea next. Then it was me, and finally your great-grandmother would help herself. She was a good cook. As she'd savor her first mouthful, she'd looked into our eyes expecting a comment. *"Buono!"* one of us would exclaim, and that was the high point of her day. Teresa had never raised a daughter, and was not prepared to wield female solidarity when I came along.

The domestic space was reconfigured as well. Grandpa Dario kept the master bedroom and reclaimed the study while Andrea moved into Dina's small bedroom and got permission to use Dario's study for his homework. I was banned from the study whose books had poisoned my imagination, and went back to the children's bedroom, now shared with *Nonna*. The study, with its phone, desk, library, sofa, and stereo, was gradually transformed into a male domain I was too shy to enter.

Our large and rather formal drawing room had been widely used when my parents entertained. Now it was a museum I looked after to keep my world stable. Its objets d'art, including Delia's beautiful china and silverware, the antique knicknack collection on display on the decorated shelves, the crystal-drop chandeliers, and the finely embroidered tablecloths were by now luxuries whose fine taste no one enjoyed. I cherished the sheer repetitiveness of the chores, the meticulous care they entailed. I also looked after the men, especially by ironing their shirts. The iron moved quickly over the backs and fronts, more carefully over the shoulders, on the seams, the overturned collar and cuffs. The sleeves were pressed and folded. A soft touch over the folded top would end the job. My efforts were often scorned, and I was rebuked for evading the higher destiny of a senator's daughter.

"What are you doing that for?" your grandpa asked one day as I was at the ironing table. "Can't you let Clara do her job?"

I kept going.

"Gaia, didn't you hear what your father said?"

More silence.

"Oh, well," *Nonna* Teresa told Dario with a shrug. "If that's what she wants," she said as your grandfather rushed out the door.

I wish I could have explained that my erotic impulses had been brutally repressed and I did not feel capable of more creative endeavors.

The sexual liberation movement had its effects also in the lives of middle-aged professionals like your grandpa. But men his age had not processed feminist ideas. Rakish types such as Delia's father, Gaspare, became their models. Just like their predecessors, the new libertines held their lovers in little consideration and were as dishonest with them as with themselves. They simply assumed that the new fashions made sexism okay. Sure, Dario's success with women was due to his charm and intelligence, as well as his social prominence as a congressman. The absence of divorce made his opportunities even greater, since he was a safer partner for an affair than a married man. Yet the rift between his public persona and private person widened with Delia gone. Being a widower cast a shadow on his public image—How did his wife die? What was the problem? What were the hidden secrets of the family? In private he was unable to live up to our expectations as a parent.

Andrea and I had been raised in a democratic family where issues were discussed out in the open and decisions were negotiated. We were trusted and learned to be trusting in return, we felt unique and complementary. After the death of your grandmother Delia, your grandpa's personal life was up for grabs. Was he going to marry again? Would we move to a different place? What about *Nonna* Teresa—would she too be part of the new household? Whatever his thoughts might have been, he certainly was not prepared to discuss his plans with us openly, nor did he intend to make us part of the decision-making process. Since our relationships were no longer based on trust and confidence, it was necessary to take control. Your great-grandpa Gaspare, Dario's father-in-law and our neighbor, observed my every move and reported on it for the supposed well-being of the family. They talked late at night, when your grandpa came home, usually over a couple of brandies, and Dario came to rely on these reports more and more. Gaspare's snitching was a form of *omertà*, a way to keep within the family information that would supposedly dishonor its men.

With his public image under control, Grandpa then proceeded to practice clandestine nonmonogamy. He did make a good-faith attempt to form a blended family with his current wife Marina. She was a sweetheart from his twenties who had returned from California after a ten-year marriage with a GI she met at the end of World War II. She had a short, plumpish body. She was feisty and energetic with her blue eyes and straight black hair. A divorcee from her American marriage, she now lived with her two children who were a bit older than

Andrea and me. Raised near the sequoia forests of Northern California, they spoke English, ate muffins and marshmallows, and looked bouncy and happy. We spent several summer vacations together, and things seemed to go well.

As the firstborn daughter of a widower, I was the inevitable "obstacle" to my father's marriage. Due to the Vatican's pervasive power, the Italian law did not allow divorces until 1974 so that this practice was virtually unknown. Second marriages lived under the shady legacy of the premature death that made them possible while Italian men were known for killing their wives with impunity to remarry younger flames, as did the Marcello Mastroianni character in *Divorce, Italian Style,* which made this practice famous also abroad.

In June 1968 Dario introduced Andrea and me to Marina. The weather had improved and we all went on a day trip to the beach. Marina was talkative, asking a lot of questions as Dario drove. Andrea and I were elated even though the beach was still windy and the white sand flew around, annoyingly. Dario felt a bit restless, as was typical when he was not "working." I figured Dario and Marina had been friends for a while, and wondered, for a moment, why I had never heard about her before. *There must be a good reason,* I thought. At the end of the day, Dario and Marina felt the trip had been a success toward the project of blending their families. Eventually, they planned summer vacations in nice beach cottages with children and friends.

Marina's children were responsible and their mother trusted them. They took hitchhiking trips with their friends, traveling to Amsterdam, Copenhagen, and Paris. I thought it would be nice if Marina and Dario got together: Then I'd be trusted again, and maybe I'd travel abroad.

Clara, the cleaning lady, was by now my best friend in the family and I told her about Marina and her kids. "They're very nice," I said as she looked at me in dismay.

"What's wrong?" I asked.

"I don't think your mother would be happy," she replied. "I believe they have been lovers for a while, maybe since before your mother got sick."

I was shaken. "Why haven't they told us? What was so wrong with me, then?" Since the uproar about Roberto, I had been getting fat and ugly to stave off men's attention. If I exercised my sexual allure, I'd be a whore. If not, a fool! Life felt safe only as the scapegoat of the family.

I remembered my mother's flirts and I used to know who they were and why they might have been interested in case she became available. How could Dario not be privy to the information? But he must not have returned the favor. I could see Delia's mind crossed by bad omens; I could hear her confront him with a question, "Is something going on?" Dario would duck. In the public mind, a man's affair only measured the extent to which his wife had failed to truly love him. But Dario knew Delia did not think this way. She'd expect him to resolve his affairs and come back to her in earnest. Yet he said nothing and allowed her to feel her trust betrayed, and now I knew this was the end of her.

One day at lunch I told Dario, "Please don't bring Marina around here again." I knew that *Nonna* Teresa would not object, but I secretly hoped Marina would demand an explanation. I wondered why no word came. Eventually, I stopped speaking to Dario altogether and the two of us stayed frozen, stubbornly, in a wordless relationship until I met your father.

When I returned from the convent, in 1971, I knew I would marry as soon as the opportunity came along. Grandpa Dario was even more flabbergasted about my second male lover than he had been about the first. My contacts with the religious institutions were forays into the humble social milieus our privileged student movement wanted to reach out to. For me this was a way to nurture a desire to better understand the world we wanted to change. For Grandpa it was simply another way to get myself in trouble. Lisandro had a clear record, but his brother had been in jail for pandering and his mother had been a prostitute. They were from those underclass milieus in Naples' underbelly where crime was a way of life and a second nature. I used to think that Lisandro's polio was a blessing for he was mildly affected, and this handicap had granted him access to education via the religious institutions that helped the poor. Unemployment was rampant, but disabled people had precedence by government policy so that a high school diploma would guarantee him a stable job. This qualified him to me as an okay date, since he'd provide basic income for our family.

Predictably, your grandfather did not see it that way. Like most people in his generation, his thinking was saturated with the idea of progress. Thanks to technological advancements, tomorrow was going to be better than yesterday and progress was going to defeat poverty, illness, and pain. Indeed, for his children, Dario had provided a more affluent childhood than the one he had. Alone, he was now faced with the new sexual ethos again, but this time the question was even more puzzling. *Why would a healthy and sound senator's daughter want to go out with the crippled orphan of a prostitute?* he must have asked himself. Of course, he did not realize that I no longer was the child of privilege I was raised as. He was still hurting for his loss and certainly not prepared to deal with my regression. Why would a young woman of good prospects so declass herself?

The sexuality of disabled persons was considered a monstrous perversity; responding to their advances was condescending if not perverse in itself. There was no understanding for the kind of unconditional love one would get. My boyfriend was tall and handsome, with an athletic body and strong muscles to compensate for his weaker leg. He was the "right" height, a bit taller than I. On one warm night in a neighborhood park, we went "all the way." I didn't find it especially pleasurable but it was a good way to get started. The smell of crushed grass mingled with the pungency of the soil as I watched the dimly lit urban skyline. We continued to be lovers for about two years. Luckily, as it turned out later, I was low on female hormones, for birth-control systems were hard to come by and men would not use condoms with a "respectable girl." But the movement had had its effect and some things were beginning to change.

At the other end of the city, a women's clinic had opened where one could get a prescription for the pill, officially sold as a headache remedy. The bus ride to the *Tiburtino* was endless. The anonymity of this blue-collar, working-class area of Rome distracted me from my fears in these furtive trips, but the pill I got turned out to have a major toxic effect. This new drug had been researched in the United States, with some brands high in male hormones and short-term tested only. Perhaps I was low on female hormones; perhaps I got a pill that had been banned by the FDA and was now being marketed overseas where its side effects were unknown. Be that as it may, after a few months I lost my period altogether. This foretold the risks of using new drugs for me, but since my body gave no signs of pregnancy I was not all that worried.

After two years with Lisandro, I came to understand how much my lover had been affected by his abusive background. He was extremely jealous, perhaps because he felt undeserving of my love, but ironically his jealousy alienated me more than his disability. He would demonstrate his love in violent ways. The *Parco dello Zodiaco,* where we first made love, was presided over by the *Madonnina,* a large statue of the Virgin colored in gold that dominates the valley below. One day he came with two small rings that were to symbolize our commitment and we put them on. Then he started to question me relentlessly as to who else I liked, was seeing or thinking of. He grabbed me by my shoulders and shook me.

"What have you been doing? Tell me! You want to dump me, right? You'd rather be with someone else!"

"No," I'd say, "not as long as you treat me well."

But then he claimed that there *was* a reason not to treat me well. "You don't make me love you because you're already thinking of someone else. You're planning your next move, aren't you? Who is he? Tell me! I've got to know!"

What I answered didn't matter for he'd not believe me. Eventually, he became so upset that he took his ring off, then got mine off also, and threw both into the bushes. Of course, there was no finding them! Shameful and helpless, he asked for my forgiveness and I gave it to him, but realized this could not go on. I had stayed in the relationship long enough to know why many women put up with violent men. Lisandro knew that Grandpa Dario used to beat me with his belt. When I told him to stop the violence or I would tell my dad, he laughed at me and said, "I'm sure *Papà* will tell you 'you made your own bed, girl, now lie in it!'" Eventually, one of your grandfather's lovers, Katia, came to my rescue.

As a widower Dario could not be monogamous because he was no longer capable of a full emotional involvement like the one he had with Delia. His classy catch had died on him, damaging his profile and emotions. He had to split his investments so that he could bear the loss. What he did not understand was that the dishonesty of these investments could in itself cause the loss he was afraid of, especially when the other person was too trusting to repay in the same way. Like Delia, Katia was such a person, and she must have noticed I was in a bad way.

Katia was a simultaneous interpreter in Italian and French, and had traveled all over the world. She was from a politically active Jewish family, and so had firsthand knowledge of exile and expatriation. She was a polyglot, and had been to many countries all by herself as a professional. She was on her second marriage, since her first had been contracted in France, where divorce was possible. Her two daughters were half-siblings, and this was not a problem with them. Katia was a confidante to both, and knew all about their sexual activities and boyfriends. She also loved to have sex with Dario and was not the least bit ashamed of it. Dario's latest scheme against Lisandro was to have the police investigate him, which only marked his powerlessness further, since at least on paper Lisandro had a clear record. There were no laws to have an abuser restricted from getting near his victim yet. Katia asked me about my sexuality in a nice, trusting way, and the floodgates flew open, "My boyfriend beats me up, and *Papà* only makes things worse. Also, I haven't had a period in almost six months already."

"Aren't you pregnant?" Katia asked, worried.

"No," I said. "At least, I don't think so. Do I look pregnant to you?"

"Well, you don't, but then, if you're not pregnant, why is your period gone? Won't we have to find out what happened to it?"

We went to her gynecologist together. The violence of which I was victim surfaced in those conversations, and suddenly I knew I deserved better. Katia was the next best thing to a support group for survivors of domestic violence I had, and I feel a deep bond to her to this day.

XIX
A Marriage of Politics

I realized Grandpa would never approve of my male lovers. As long as I was enthralled with the guy, Dario hated his guts. His hostility often helped to bring my relationships to an end, after which he started to have some respect for the unlucky fellow. "I don't know what she finds in him," he confessed to Katia one day. When I met your father Giulio your grandfather Dario didn't even seem to notice what an improvement he was. He wanted jurisdiction over my choices as if he was going to bed the fellow himself. Was he afraid that some day I would discover men weren't necessary? I thought he'd approve of a lover who was my peer, both culturally and intellectually. But that scared the shit out of me. *"Why?"* Grandpa must have thought, *"Hasn't her mother been happy?"* But as a child, I had seen what my father missed. Your grandmother Delia did not live on to enjoy the concordance she and Dario had. As soon as they had children, her career became secondary; her desires were crushed and he absorbed her intellectual energy. When he left school for politics, she supported him, but when her opportunity came to get into educational TV, it did not occur to him that it would have been as important for him to support her. Finally, when it came to purchasing a family home, he encouraged her to accept her father's offer. My grandfather too wanted his daughter near him, and Delia found herself stuck between two men. The patriarchal order surrounded her—the cancer she got was a natural way to smother a flame that had been asphyxiated already. A lover my father would approve of would be one with the potential to behave like him, and I felt this would be a deadly trap for me. If I found him, how would I stave off the pressure to make him the center of my life? And if I allowed that to happen, how would I ever find a center of my own?

In my situation marriage was both dangerous and necessary. It was dangerous because if I married the "right" person, circumstances would conspire to turn me into a satellite in the life of another. It was necessary because the status of being married would temporarily grant me a center of gravity of my own. So when I found an acceptable partner, I went ahead.

Your father, Giulio, and I met in Sardinia on a summer vacation, in 1974. Grandpa, Andrea, and I had company, for our second cousin Silvia joined us for the vacation. She was an eighteen-year old brunette with a cute body and a sweet face. We were staying at Turas, that beautiful, dilapidated hotel on the island's west coast, where the Mediterranean is still clean and transparent. We had been told about the nearby town of Bosa, where your father vacationed with his family—a town frozen in a pre-modern age, still on the estuary of the river Temo. As we traveled, I observed the azure river meandering slowly into the bay, and how people grew their vegetables near its red-clay bed. To the south side, a wild plateau lined the river canyon. Opposite was the hill with the old town, accessed through a stone bridge of a light-sienna red fading into purple. A medieval castle topped the old town, its alleys paved in cobblestone.

Silvia's modest demeanor, dark hair, and full bosom made her very feminine. Naturally, the local guys got word of the two female strangers, and came to check us out right away. Gavino, Antonio, and your father, Giulio, seemed to me *dolce vita* types modeled on Fellini's *vitelloni,* looking for antidotes to the snug monotony of provincial life. They spent their vacations in Bosa, while the nearby city of Tattari, in the north of the island, was their main residence. They were older than us and more established. Gavino was a schoolteacher and a visual artist; with a beard, he looked solemn, an intellectual. Antonio, nearsighted, with a dark moustache and long hair, had some kind of governmental job. An extrovert, he looked somewhat disillusioned, expended. Your father was fun and seemed more responsible, with a slender body and pianist hands. There was something incongruous about him, which he liked to draw attention to. His ash-brown hair was thin and wavy, while his moustache was bristly and red. He'd let people touch it to find out how stiff it was.

"My pubic hair is like this too, in case you'd like to know," he'd laugh away.

All three were eager to demonstrate proverbial Sardinian hospitality by taking us all over the island on explorations. They each drove funny cars, such as your dad's plastic jeep from Citroen that we still had when you were born. On the backseat they carried the most important guest, *il bambino,* an open bottle of gin or brandy wrapped in some cloth like a baby. I have to say that this bundle of joy seemed to be their most cherished possession!

The shrubbery that covered the plateaus of northern Sardinia was good pasture for abundant sheep and goats whose milk made wonderful *pecorino* and goat cheese. The landscape looked pristine as if devoid of human presence, typical for this depopulated island, but new for us from "the Continent." It had the eeriness and premonition of Apache land. At the center of the island was the region of Barbagia, famous for its brigands and rebels who stole livestock and kidnapped children for ransom from the local landowners. We visited its capital, Orgosolo, home of Graziano Mesina, the bandit whose legend inspired many leaders in the *movimento.* As we traveled with our new friends, we realized what the local custom was. The group would make one stop at each bar that lined the main avenue in a town, or *corso.* The stop was over when every male in the group had paid for a round of drinks. Women, considered lightweights, accepted a chocolate kiss instead. The bars smelled of *acquavite* and had standing room only.

"Whatcha'll getting?" Antonio asked.

"A whiskey," Gavino answered.

"A gin and tonic for me," your father added.

"A brandy," one of the local fellows who had joined the party said.

"I pass," I heard Andrea's voice say.

"You can't," Antonio insisted.

"Please."

"No way!"

"A martini then."

"Now we're talking. And you gals?" Antonio asked Silvia and me.

"A soda and a chocolate kiss."

There were seven bars on Orgosolo's *corso,* and several local fellows joined the group, which explains why your uncle Andrea ended up bent over a nearby tree's lower branch, vomiting.

The hills near the windy roads were speckled with dead car bodies, I noticed the next day. As I looked on, our hosts hastened to lay the blame on the roads.

"The government never gets around to building us good high-ways," Gavino said.

"How come that car ended up all the way over there?" I asked, pointing to the body of a car down the hill from a steep turn.

Your dad's moustache curled as he made a knowing face, but I didn't know enough about alcoholism to understand what was going on.

Giulio looked both at home and out of place in the dry landscape. He picked up the tabs and made sure my driver was sober. He was the age of most leaders in the student movement, but had not partici-pated for he lived far away—yet the "revolution" had affected him. He was getting out of a shotgun marriage arranged to legitimize his first baby, your half sister Aurelia, and out of a drunk-driving acci-dent that landed him in the hosptial for thirty-six days. "I was a passenger," he told me.

He must have gotten himself in trouble trying to practice the freer world we preached, I thought. Paternity could be recognized only through mar-riage even when the parents split before the child was born. Abortion was a crime and there was no divorce.

"I made Anna pregnant by accident," he explained as he drove, "and married her after the baby was born. She lived with her mom—they're independently wealthy. I stayed at her place for a couple of days then ran back home—but we're friends."

Perhaps it was his vulnerability, perhaps his dainty body, but he felt very androgynous and feminine—someone a bisexual-to-be could easily love.

The six of us stayed together throughout the vacation, and I no-ticed Giulio always made sure I rode next to him. On the last evening, my hand brushed against his face as he drove over the last stretch of the road. We were back from our Barbagia trip at 5 a.m., exhausted and happy. Grandpa Dario was up waiting for us.

"Where were you?" he asked as he slapped my face.

No answer.

"Go up and pack your bags," he ordered us. "We have a ferry to catch tomorrow."

Andrea and Silvia rushed upstairs and I followed.

"He has been up all night," the hotel manager mumbled with a knowing face.

"I can't wait for this to be over," Dario told him, rolling his eyes. "Thank god we're going home."

In the middle of our vacation, your grandpa had had to fly back to Rome for Italian terrorism had struck again. It was the bomb on the *Italicus* train, which killed twelve. Congress had been summoned in an emergency. He barely made it back before the vacation was over. We scoffed at his fury as our friends drove away, Giulio's fingers clasping the stubble I stroked.

There must have been a promise in that gesture, since a few weeks later your dad came to the "Continent" for a visit. Your grandfather Dario was too busy to keep tabs on me, and *Nonna* Teresa summered in Fosca. Giulio and I couldn't wait to be on our own. Traveling was a political imperative for we responded to terrorism by not allowing it to keep us home. We first did it in a small, triangular tent, while in Bologna at the *Festa dell'Unità,* the popular-culture festival sponsored by the largest political force in the Italian left, the Partito Comunista. I could not have thought of a better way to evade parental surveillance than participating in this event. Bologna, with its old towers sticking out of the haze in the Po River delta, was about 300 hundred miles to the north of Rome. It was the capital of the left, with its festival in a vast lowland area outside the city walls. It was damp and I remember our skins swished with sweat as we lay down on the floor.

"Why don't you take that off?" your dad said as he pulled on my soaking shirt.

I lay down, the air moist with our body scents. On our skins the sweat melted with our juices wrapping us in their wetness.

This first encounter vibrated with the political tensions of the day, but as the fervor tapered off we had sex in many places, including the kitchen, the study, the car, various bedrooms. Yet your father did not like nature, and I never managed to have sex with him in the open air. I had not discovered the woman-on-top position yet, and was left to my own devices when he came first.

In the queer flashbacks of my marriage, Giulio presented the manufacture of gender in unexpected ways. The mirror he held up to my face reflected the pieces of my fragmented self. I'm in my twenties, a bit wimpy and embarrassed. I sit on the roadside in downtown Bosa. It's Mardi Gras and I watch the man I am going to marry march in full drag-queen attire at the local parade. Giulio wears heavy make up, a wig, a sluttish miniskirt, and high pumps. His briskly red moustache matches the long Italian sausage tied to his waist, in full view between his legs. His friend Luigi walks at his side in a black tuxedo. Both smile, their round eyes glowing in a drunken haze. The female impersonator suffers from a mysterious ailment. He whines, *"Ahi, sa golza!"* (Ouch, my crotch!). I observe Giulio's small shoulders, heart-shaped lips, and perfectly well-rounded legs. *He'd make a cute girlfriend,* I think, *but I couldn't sport her around because I'm not a man.* Cross-dressing was very common in Bosa, where the traditions of a premodern, quasi-pagan carnival still held sway. I was both attracted and repelled by them.

Your father had a limited interest in sex, or heterosex, I should say. Between us sex usually happened when he was tipsy enough to let his guard down but not quite drunk yet. I had the impression that one had to catch him at the right moment—distracted from the bottle he assiduously courted with his male friends—and lure him away before his desire would drown into the booze. He didn't have a lot of imagination, but was never violent or obnoxious in any way.

It was January 1976, and I was going to turn twenty-two in September. Giulio had been holding down a stable job with a Sardinian bank since the days of the shotgun marriage. When we began to go steady, he transferred to its Rome branch. He rented a nice apartment and was responsible for himself. But he became involved with the union and was immediately sent back to Sardinia. I often stayed with him and wanted to continue to do so, even if this implied getting further away from my family. He didn't want to go back to his parents' home. There were only two ways to get married: A Catholic church wedding would get us automatically registered with the Italian state, and its religious bond would be indissoluble; the other option was a civil wedding. Italy was becoming more secular than in my parents' days, and civil weddings were acceptable. But neither your dad nor I cared for any kind of wedding, and so, when he was transferred back, I packed my things and kept my bags ready.

"I'll move to Sardinia as soon as he has a place to stay," I bravely told my dad.

Tattari was a small city and rental apartments for unmarried couples were not easy to come by.

"But we mean business and my parents know," Giulio reassured me on the phone.

Your grandfather Dario called your other grandparents. "I want her to leave home with the proper papers."

But your dad's shotgun marriage had been celebrated in church.

"Only the Vatican can dissolve it," your other grandfather said, "but maybe I can pull my strings and get him an annulment." And he did.

Your other grandparents are Catholics, and a civil wedding would have offended them. So we settled for a church wedding.

The somewhat basic sex your father and I practiced worked off and on until our wedding day. I remember our "first night," in a room with antique furniture and beige plaster walls. I wore the embroidered nightgown of *Nonna* Teresa. Your father's slender body left his striped pajamas half empty. We lay down and felt strange, out-of-place characters in a trite play.

We had somewhat caved in to societal pressures, but stood our ground in a way. Unlike my mother, I was not a virgin, and unlike my father, Giulio encouraged his former and current wives to get along.

"Gaia, meet Anna," he said one day when we were all at Tattari's central café.

"Hello." She smiled and put out her hand.

We sat down and they ordered drinks. The camaraderie between them was noticeable.

"He makes a good friend, but not a great husband, I'm afraid," she whispered as he paid.

The first of three brothers in his family, Giulio had been raised like a "true boy," and was inept at all household chores. But he was not jealous, and there was a gentle, feminine edge about him, waiting to be discovered.

A few months after the wedding, we started to have sex on the rhythm-method in reverse for I wanted to get pregnant and had had my hormone level raised.

"There is something repressive about being married," I observed, "but while I'm at it, I might as well get my reproductive job done right away."

"I'm not sure I'm ready," Giulio said, yet did not oppose my plan.

My body ached for pregnancy, perhaps because I was afraid I'd turn sterile from chemical contraceptives. And as I did get pregnant with you, my baby, my body was absorbed in the bliss of its own plenitude—a self-generated state of erotic ecstasy.

As my belly grew, so did the women's movement in Italy and its pressure for a law that would decriminalize abortion and make that widespread practice safer. Many women had lost their lives in back-alley abortions, and, for all we know, their pregnancies could have started in rape, since a married woman could never say no. I had never had an abortion, but had heard about the mother of Andrea's friend Ivan, who had been killed in a back-alley abortion when her kids weren't even teenagers yet. Many doctors practiced abortion at home, but sometimes a woman's uterus would rupture in the process, and one would hesitate to go to the hospital for fear of getting caught. That's how Ivan's mother had bled to death at the age of thirty-six.

This woman I never met was only trying to raise her kids and protect her body from an unexpected tenant. How could I not feel that legal and safe abortions were really necessary? Not a substitute for birth control, abortion was an extreme remedy, and the new law, the famous *Legge 194,* permitted it only up to the twelfth week of pregnancy. But its opponents organized a referendum for its repeal with the support of the Catholic Church. I felt it was important for us women to keep this option in place—that we women would not have to risk our lives if our birth-control systems failed.

The *Partito Comunista* embraced the abortion cause. A general election was coming up and I was in midpregnancy. In Sardinia, where some features of a premodern culture still held sway, the body of a pregnant woman was sacred. The best foods were administered to her. Her wish was everybody else's command, since people believed that a pregnant woman's unfulfilled yearnings would result in a birthmark on the baby, of the color of the craved aliment. I was a part-time student at the local university, and a homemaker. The city of Tattari was a swing-voter area and abortion was a warhorse of the left, for they knew women wanted to defend the law, as they had done earlier with divorce laws. The headquarters of the campaign was at the local Communist Party cell. The largest political formation of the left, the PCI was both progressive enough to embrace the impulses of the women's movement, and strong enough to wield the political leverage necessary to make good on them. I spent most of my spare time at the cell.

The main element in my casual attire was a blue cotton skirt that folded like a wallet over my pregnant belly. Its strings tied in a bow, which I remember adjusting to your size, my beloved growing abdominal tenant.

"You make a perfect ad for the point we want to make," a comrade said. "We're out to protect life and the women who choose to give it, not to 'kill babies'."

At rallies and demonstrations I helped to distribute information sporting my swollen belly to persuade law-abiding citizens to defend a woman's right to control what happens in her abdomen. In popular mythology, communists were heathen ogres who ate babies, red devils who'd land you in hell. The party in power, Democrazia Cristiana, was a centrist conservative formation that had traditionally benefited from red scares. But thanks to the women who knew that reproductive choice matters, the elections went well. The Partito Comunista tallied its adversary by only two percentage points, 35 to 37. It was the biggest victory of the Italian left throughout the 1970s, and would lead to the famous *Compromesso Storico,* a popular-front type of agreement between majority and opposition on a program negotiated together. I was proud to contribute to a political change that empowered women who took our reproductive process into our hands. Your father, who as you know was not from a political family, was very supportive and participated as well.

XX
Quagmires

I remember my pregnancy with you as a time of elation no desire ever perturbed, which ended in violent childbirth. You, my beloved tenant, must have been happy, since I had never felt so well before, and since getting you out of there was so unpleasant. I loved to dance with you in my big belly. In Tattari, one gave birth at the hospital, for the midwife system had been wiped out by modern medicine. I was so absorbed in my tantric joy the night before my water broke that I wanted to go to a dance party at a country house accessed by an unpaved road. Perhaps my body was so afraid of the hospital that it wanted to run away. Your dad ignored me and insisted we stay home. Then he drove me to the maternity guard. I remember a twelve-hour night of labor alone in the guard's hallway looking at the shaft of an unused elevator. The nurses were playing cards and wouldn't hear my calls. No one even looked at my birth canal or measured my dilation. Then the delivery room filled with angry voices. It was 5 a.m. The doctor got up and realized I was ready. I lay supine on the stretcher. He and the nurse jumped over my stomach and pushed over my belly. A big cut over the lower vaginal labia and wall, a strong pull of the forceps, and finally they managed to get your head out of there. The doctor sowed his stitches over my live flesh, and then sent me away as one who didn't "push well." For years I fantasized of getting even with him in the Lorena Bobbitt way.

I am in the hospital bed with newborn you on my lap in an outfit I've patiently knitted. I look bloated and my butt aches with my weight over my sewn groin. My body and yours are not connecting in a healthy way. Babies are kept in a separate room and when the nurse brings you in my milk surge is gone. I give you my breast. You suck but there's not much to be had. Then you're taken away and you drink from a bottle. The next time you come in it's even worse. That body-to-body connection through the breast and the milk flow never happens. Giulio's mother sees that and wants to help.

"In my time children were born at home. I breast-fed my three boys for years," she says as she helps me change clothes and puts clean towels in my drawer. I hear my first adult feminist sentence: "You must be happy you have a girl!"

"Why?"

Your father's mother leans close to my ear. "She'll be your friend. You'll have more company."

It was not the best childbirth, but I was proud to beat the system and have you, my baby.

"It's a good thing the doctor sewed you tight," the nurse said. "Your vagina will return to normal, and you won't get prolapse of the uterus later on."

You were a fragile, minute little baby, with green eyes like your father's dad. Luckily, the forceps did not damage you even though your face was red with birth trauma. You must have liked to live in my belly just as much as I liked having you in there. I didn't know what an episiotomy was, nor that it would take years for me to enjoy vaginal sex again.

In the summer of 1977, when you were only five months old, we moved back to Rome. It was Giulio's decision, but Rome was my hometown and I did not oppose it. We rented a spacious apartment in a terraced *palazzina* at the top of a hill, a private garden on the back, and a nice condominium front lawn. My grandfather's lover—the woman who watched TV with him in his old days and after being the cause of my grandmother Angela's separation—was the one who helped me find this gem in the tight rental market of those days, blocked by noneviction policies and rental controls. She lived downstairs, and I could see her children play in the garden. I wondered if it was true that her marriage was a front for her relation with your great-grandfather, as it was rumored in the family. The youngsters I saw from my balcony were about my age and their aquiline profile was modeled on Gaspare's hooked nose—the dreaded shape I had wanted to avoid by marrying your Sardinian father. Maybe they were my half-cousins after all.

The living room looked over the valley in which the historical center of the city lay. One could see St. Peter's dome. We had a nearby bus stop, walking-distance stores, and other amenities. Giulio and I slowly resumed our sex lives together, but having sex hurt terribly, at least in the conventional way. Occasionally, something exciting would happen between us in bed, but we didn't pursue it for fear of being judged or manipulated by each other.

As we settled back in the capital, our lives started to move in different directions. Raised to speak Italian and French, I had a dormant French persona inside and she was pressing for expression. Your father seemed locked in his own world. I tried to interest him in my studies, but he didn't respond. I didn't know what was wrong. We spent way more than we had, and by the fifteenth we'd be broke. Was the money really not enough, or did your father spend too much on drinks and partying with friends? I tried to have him stick to the budget, but before I knew it, his mom would slip money into his hands. A whole gang of neighborhood friends hung out at our home. I entertained them so they wouldn't spend money in bars and restaurants. Once I brought two large bottles of aquavit from Sardinia. This extract from vine branches was illegal and had 90 percent alcohol. I hoped it would quench their thirst. But one night a semipermanent guest broke the bottle and spilled the contents on the floor. No one bothered to apologize to me.

You were growing up in a world full of uncertainties. After the numerous attacks against the civil population, terrorist forces were taking on the big guys. Prime Minister Aldo Moro had been kidnapped by the Red Brigades. He was the promoter of the *Compromesso Storico,* the "Historical Compromise" which Grandpa Dario had mediated from his independent position within the left. Grandpa felt threatened. Violence was taking over at the expense of negotiation and things were getting out of control. The debate became parochial and everybody blamed anybody except themselves. I felt my future must be somewhere else, and began to listen to the urge to meet more bilingual, bicultural persons. I wanted you, my baby, to be part of that as well.

My queering moments became triangulated. In Rome I was a stay-at-home mom, in Tattari a part-time student, a guest at Giulio's parents, and I discovered that commuting between these two was a great way to have affairs. I met Gino on the ferry from Sardinia to the "Continent." He had lived in Paris and his revolutionary allure awoke my dormant erotic energies. We made love at his place in Tattari. He had more experience and was sensitive to the fact that my vagina was out of commission. He gave me oral sex for the first time and the stimulation opened my birth channel up eventually. Then he disappeared for a while, until one night, in Rome, I found myself in bed with him and a stained-glass artist who claimed to be his best friend. They wanted to share me in a three-way. But they soon realized I was not prepared for that spontaneous erotic play, and one night they stood me up near the old prison of Regina Coeli, where I learned to depend on the kindness of strangers. A man stopped his car to talk to me and I jumped in to go to his apartment and make love. He was from the Middle East and lived in LA. I practiced my English, being present to the moment, and attaching no strings to sex. My erotic presence was more intense because there were no future plans—behaving like one of the guys empowered me. Having sex in a foreign language was exciting as well, and my lover, who was visiting Rome, kept a very nice memory of me, as he repeatedly wrote in his notes.

In the meantime, as I discovered later, Giulio kept carrying on with our au pair from England, Melanie. She had been hired with the twin purpose of babysitting and helping me with English fluency, in view of my upcoming fourth-level exams. I was getting close to writing my senior thesis, and was disappointed that Giulio, who wouldn't take an interest in my literary efforts, stole the attention of my British au pair instead. I remembered my grandfather and Delia's pretty French au pairs. Italian men still had a special thing for *le straniere,* the north European women whose paradises of sexual freedom they craved.

As a young woman now married, I had returned to the educational system with good intentions, even though I was aware that it did not promote a person's creative intelligence, and even as I already felt it was not prepared to help me learn about myself or those like me. The knowledge that was presented as valuable before me was all about men. As a literature major, I was aware of the few texts by women about which one was supposed to know. But by and large, the writers who counted were male, and female writers existed only for the purpose of adjoining them to one another in a convincing story. In the Italian system, all knowledge in the humanities was framed as historical and was taught in a master narrative that corresponded to the story about themselves that cultured, straight, European men passed as universal history. One did not study literature per se, but "the history of literature." I sensed that the his/story of literature the Italian university system presented as that which there was to know was a body of knowledge that did not include me. This made me feel expendable, and I looked for a position from which to recuperate a portion of that self-knowledge to which I aspired in a still quite obscure way.

But given the situation, studying works by female authors was an option beyond the pale. All university professors were males mostly unaware of the fact that women wrote. Besides, the system controlled knowledge by failing to provide libraries that gave access to the books professors ignored. How could a student make her case? Fortunately, professors could not ignore the fact that female characters were written into canonical works. As a result, these representations of women by men were the most feminist objects of study one could possibly work on. For a *Laurea* thesis, a professor would assign a student a topic. An exceedingly democratic professor would sometimes allow a promising student to propose a topic of her own, always based on an author the professor claimed expertise on. I learned about the Irish playwright Sean O'Casey from one of my professors, Giuseppe Serpillo, who liked Irish literature and became my director. I asked to analyze the development of female characters in his plays and he agreed. My urge to find a focus related to my embodiment must have come across in a powerful way. My first love for women was eminently literary, and it didn't even remotely occur to me that, when the peels of my homo- and biphobic upbringing would come off, this intellectual love would also become spiritual and erotic.

For a short while, my relationship with Giulio was revived by our affairs. I was more lubricated and loving and, eventually, I became pregnant again—except I was not sure who the father was. Giulio came to Tattari with you and I for graduation and we stayed with your grandparents, in the six-story building where Gino's relatives lived as well. One day as I was going out with him and you, my baby, Gino entered the elevator we were riding. Your dad looked at Gino who returned the gaze and both seemed to giggle under their moustaches.

"Maybe the Tattari grapevine has worked and Giulio knows already," I thought. I pictured what would happen if the new baby looked like Gino and made up my mind to terminate the pregnancy. Abortion had been decriminalized and was now accessible free of charge at county hospitals. But things were uncertain, for many physicians refused to practice it based on conscientious objection, which crowded the system causing delays and made me decide to go to a private abortionist instead.

The idea of a marriage successfully ending with both spouses alive was new. The women's movement introduced the concept in the wake of the sexual revolution, and a divorce law had been approved in the early 1970s, confirmed by referendum in 1974. The sexual freedom we had experimented with was followed by a reformist agenda that upgraded the lay institution of marriage and put it on a par with its religious competitor. The Vatican routinely annulled the Catholic marriages of those who could afford it or were well connected, with no provision for child support. Your father's first marriage was an example, which was annulled by the Church as nonconsummated even though a child had been born. Ironically, atheists had to stay married for all eternity, for lay marriages, not under the jurisdiction of the Church, could never be dissolved according to the law. Many free unions developed out of marriages that were de facto dissolved. Divorce was presented as the policy that would allow them to end, therefore turning free unions into new marriages. The approved law carried alimony provisions and a waiting-period clause, designed to avoid impulsive divorces. In a no-fault case, five years had to go by before a legally separated spouse could apply for divorce. This period was later cut down to three years, but if one of the partners opposed divorce, it could be prolonged indefinitely.

My marriage with your father was caught in the quagmire of the waiting-period clause. For me, the time to break away came after graduation, in 1980, when I had been holding down a full-time job in the tourist industry for a few months. There was no open job market, so I had enlisted Grandpa Dario's help to get a job through his political connections, and I was now able to provide for myself. But that's when the inequalities between your father and I came to the fore. We were now a two-income family and should have been better off. But even though I had a university education, I made less money than he did. He felt all common expenses should be divided equally, even though he had a better pay—he could keep more spending money that way. As a student I had accepted my role of homemaker because students didn't get paid, now I felt we should share chores since both of us had eight-to-five jobs. He was not prepared to clean, cook, or parent, except when I forced the issue and left him alone with you, my baby. Ironically, he did take good care of you, except he'd not admit it was his job nor that he enjoyed it. Now we could afford some babysitting, and found a nice girl, Sandra, who was young and affectionate, unobtrusive and very patient. But Giulio distracted her and called attention to himself.

As I became more involved with my job, being married to your father came to look as a sacrifice that had no purpose. Our personal relationship seemed to have dissolved, our home life was unrewarding, and there were no recreational or cultural activities we enjoyed together. Of course, there was you, my baby, but there, too, I felt he was using you to make me feel less than a good parent, and thus keep me under his control.

Eventually, I decided to move on. Our marriage had not survived our silly affairs and we got a legal separation, which became your longtime affliction and our parents.' Divorce was new in Italy and there was no socially accepted way to process it, which earned me the stigma of the bad spouse who "broke the home."

As the years went by, my move to California put an ocean and a continent between your father and me, which made divorce both impracticable and superfluous. As a result, the limbo our dissolving family was in became permanent. Your dad and I were legally separated for a total of eighteen years, during which our families mediated the tensions this quagmire created. I had your legal custody and could have claimed alimony, but Giulio had vowed to support you only when you were with him or his family. I knew he'd keep his word and was forced to give you up to them eventually. In the effort to be good grandparents, my dad and his parents made up for our shortcomings, and learned to know and respect each other in the process.

When I finished graduate school, in 1987, my ambiguous status at the registry mirrored my confusing citizenship situation. Just as I was a married person out of my marriage but still not quite able to marry someone else, so I was an Italian citizen out of Italy but still not quite able to establish my citizenship in the United States. My predicament as your parent was ironic as well. Getting citizenship through marriage, fake or not, would have cost me your custody, for your father would have claimed it had I filed for divorce from abroad. Keeping you with me would have made me unable to become a citizen on my own, for I could not have competed on the job market as a free and single person.

The quagmire caught my parenting efforts as well. As an "orphan" I had ached to become a very young parent: I wanted a good chance to see you, my offspring, grow. I also wanted to pass my mother's spiritual freedom and love for the body over to you, my dear descendant, but unlike my mother, I was not a specialized pedagogue. While I did have a rather precise sense of how to create that space, I did not have the means or authority to be the parent I wanted to be. I raised you uninterruptedly for the first four and a half years of your life, from 1977 to 1981. I took pride in being first to touch the palms of your little hands and feet. I felt the pristine texture of that skin surface and observed the designs the palm lines formed together. I tried to imagine what they meant, and how they would persist when those little limbs would be grown.

XXI
Baby

You grew up as a rather uninhibited baby. In 1977 you were a toddler at only five months old and walked before turning one. You were diminutive and delicate, with a small bone structure and thin, ubiquitous fingers just like your dad. You looked like Giulio a lot, with wide eyes, the tiniest little nose, heart-shaped lips, and a round face. There was something funky and comical about you. You did not break things or get hurt, but were adventurous in your movements and curious in your demands, and therefore were a lot of work. You were always inquisitive and daring, with a persistent desire to learn and I allowed you to make as much progress as your natural curiosity granted. I potty trained you at one and a half years old, spending about fifteen days on the project. And at two you could eat our food elegantly already, at the dining table and with a knife and fork. We were off to a good start, but I did not have the time or help to do it all my own way. At some point it became apparent that I was not going to embrace the role of mother to the point of becoming transparent—of no longer having a life of my own. Then I began to feel some criticism, especially from the women in your father's family.

I had the model of my mother in mind, Delia, but she was not there to demonstrate it or to protect me from social blame. Even though, conventionally, childrearing was supposed to totally absorb a woman's life energy, for me your birth was an incentive to desire and do more—study, work, find my own centeredness, give my life a meaning of its own. A mother's abjection had been natural for the women in your father's family, and since I did not have it, your other grandmother and her sisters gradually stepped in. In the summer months the family spent in Bosa, they took a fair share of responsibility in the child-rearing process, and they also took a large portion of your trust and affection. To make their own job easier, they instilled in you a fair amount of fear and repression I wish they would have kept to them-selves.

Sometimes they would alert me to possible baby health problems I was not aware of. One evening at a wedding when you were a few months old I was dancing with you in my arms. Giulio's mother and her sister noticed that you were a bit pale and asked if your bowel movements were regular.

"It's a bit runny," I answered.

"She must have diarrhea. For how long?"

"A few days."

"Haven't you done anything?"

"Well, I thought it would pass."

"You must give her rice water," they explained. The summer was hot. "She can get quite dehydrated."

Most of the time the advice was just a way to help me do a better job, but their apprehension disturbed me, since I thought I didn't need any help. But sometimes there was more. One summer we took our vacations in Fosca, in the large mountain house that had belonged to *Nonna* Teresa who had already passed away. Her second daughter-in-law was prematurely dying, of cancer also, and "I don't want to re-member it," she told me the last time I visited her. Your paternal grandparents joined us. You were about three years old and could climb and walk. But the staircase going down to the cellar was dark with high, irregular steps. "You can do it, Sara," I would tell you while standing behind you as you climbed on all fours. It was a way to empower you while being safe. But Giulio's mother thought you were too small and I should pick you up. I felt this would instill a useless fear in you. One evening we didn't manage to agree on what to do at the bottom of the stairs, and then I climbed first. You followed, with your grandma just behind you. But this time—perhaps your grandma's apprehension distracted you—you fell. You broke your left forearm bone, and we had to take you to the hospital for a cast, remember? It was not a bad or dangerous injury, just part of a normal growing-up process—testing the boundaries and learning to measure one's strength. Surely, it would have been better to avoid your fall. But then eventu-ally it became constructed as the result of my negligence, and you lost trust in me. I resented being regarded as a negligent parent when in fact I had only tried to empower you to learn. Eventually, I understood that sharing responsibilities meant sharing methods, and hoped to, at some point, successfully intercept the process of programming you into a new female who would expect her mother to become abject for her, and would end up expecting that of herself as well when your own turn came along.

Yet those older women in your father's family must have known that things were changing, for, when I asked to take a trip on my own as a reward for my graduation, they offered to take care of you. I went to Ireland and visited the home of the playwright I wrote about, Sean O'Casey, and had a brief love affair on the way. At my return, I decided it was time your father and I broke up. My friend Veronica knew I was having trouble, and opened her home to you and me, which was okay with her family. You remember Veronica in her thirties, outspoken and energetic, with a handsome chest and bouncy legs. Her sunny expression and generous body reminded me of my mother and I felt mothered at her place. But of course that was temporary, and a few weeks later you and I moved back to my father's place. Grandpa Dario had moved out to live with Marina now his wife, but uncle Andrea was still there and was determined not to become a father figure to you. He never shared meals with us, and gave the impression that he'd rather live in a chldfree place. I felt the pressure to give him space and even looked for rental apartments, but was very well aware that my paycheck would barely cover the rent. Your great-grandfather Gaspare's apartment next door was empty, for he was in the hospital, with few chances for recovery. "Could I use it?" I asked. The answer was no. I held my ground and stayed. At night, when you were in bed, I worked on my graduate-school applications—a maze I navigated secretly and by myself.

In some ways, my relationship with you, my baby, reflected my experience of bringing you into the world. There was joy and playfulness in your explorative efforts, and I watched over them with excitement. This reminded me of your period as a happy camper in my abdomen. But at times I felt you became too much of a center of your own.

There was no room for me to continue to grow. At times you and I played like two little girls. This made me happy because as a child I longed to have a younger and more playful mother who was more of a little girl than Delia had been for me. But at times the energy in the field between you and I froze. I now see that the memory of your painful birth was in the way. The narrowness of my birth channel, the anxiety of my labor, your effort in moving forward, the pain of being temporarily stuck in there, the frustration of matching a fed suckling baby with an empty breast—all those violent interactions caused bruises in our auras that had not been healed yet. I remembered Delia explaining how it was more painful to deliver one's first baby, and I thought of Andrea, who had always been more cuddly than I was. I wanted to be a mom whose body one could jump all over, whose hair one could mess up, whose clothes one could wrinkle and smudge over. Yet I had a memory of coldness, as if my own aura reminded my mother's body of some pain. I was proud of my ecstatic pregnancy, of my body's perfect hospitality to you, my baby tenant. But now I wished I had done more to prepare for the birth. I tried to hide those unpleasant memories from myself and you, my baby, but I was not aware of the aural energy work necessary to get the job done.

In time, I was to observe that the gap in the physical relationship between myself and you, my baby, was gradually being filled by my male partners. There was some Oedipal attraction, and the curves along which desire traveled were shaped by a heterosexual social order. I worried that you would always prefer men and I gradually realized this was unfair to mothers of girls, who would never feel like a favorite parent. I felt there was a misogynist intent in the way in which the medical system handled childbirth. If mothers hated it, there was another reason for boys to be favored. I kept going back to what your father's mother told me, that I was lucky to have a girl. But you seemed to guess my dilemma, baby. *"Mamma,"* you asked over and over, "are you happy I am a girl?" I kept saying, "Yes, yes I am, yes I am, dear, yes I am" but within myself I kept wondering *why this question?* I was anxious. *Can I truly be her favorite parent?*

XXII
Erotic Lessons

It was high time I learned to become a good lover. Other than having you in my pregnant, ecstatic belly, sexuality was still my only access to the sacred—to the kind of life energy that made me feel connected with the universe. But my love stories were still monogamous and monosexual, for I still bought into the conventional dream of romantic love. The months around the separation between me and your dad were filled with friendly technical experiments that became useful later on.

During my trip to Ireland in 1980 I got my first break. I planned this study-related vacation with two friends from Sardinia, Annalisa and Simonetta. It was after my graduation, in 1979, and we were going to visit the birthplace of Sean O'Casey, the author whose plays I discussed in my *laurea* thesis. The whole voyage was especially erotic because I was inspired by the desire to connect the reality of my research with the colors, sounds, smells, gestures, and faces I had first encountered as literary. With our daily routines left behind, we became more contemplative and poetic. It was the first time we left home with only female company, and we were going to a foreign land, which I always felt gave my aura a special glow. I could sense the energy centers I later came to know as chakras open up to receive new cosmic forces. The twin excitement of freedom and novelty widened these openings and allowed in a more intense energy flow. The colors looked brighter, and a sense of magic accompanied us.

As we traveled together again, to Paris, Prague, and other destinations over our summer vacations, erotic experiments became a part of our plans, since my girlfriends and I counted on the allure of being foreigners, and on the unpredictability of traveling by train, to score at least one little fling or *storia* for each trip. We acted as confidantes to each other, and were totally complicit with one another in making things happen, even though we were fully aware of each other's more permanent emotional involvements and obligations. It was a way to practically benefit from the dissemination of the new cultural models of women's liberation, and get to know the world in a more profound and erotically engaged way. It is ironic to me now that we never thought of giving each other the sexual attention we were seeking from foreign men. Eventually, Simonetta admitted to me that perhaps we were simply cowards, but another reason was that to each other we were not enough "foreign."

From the trip to Ireland, I had to return earlier because of you, my baby, and my day job. With my girlfriends staying on, and my body-mind opened up by the multiple stimulations, on my way back I made friends with Johannes, a graduate student from UC Berkeley on his way to visit his German-Swiss family. He was a linguist, much in character with his national background and preparation. On the boat over the Channel we spoke French and he complimented me on it. We decided to stop in Paris. It was love at first sight, beautiful and innocent and intense, with no future, which only made it more authentic. Our stopover turned into an intense erotic experience that lasted for two nights and two days. We got to explore each other's bodies in their smallest details, learned their respective erotic mechanisms and played with them to the very last inkling of our energy. I finally got to try the woman-on-top position and learned to relish clitoral stimulation. I discovered his erogenous areas around the anus, and he discovered them also. This excellent sex was a productive exchange of energy that involved a total and miraculous connection of all our chakras. It helped my life take a new direction, as, one year later, in 1981, I left my life as a single parent trapped in an eight-to-five job, to move to the Western edge of the "New World."

My lessons in eroticism continued as I settled in my ambiguous status at the registry. Still in Rome, while living at my family home with you and Andrea, I was neither single nor divorced, and this limbo turned out to be my window of opportunity for experimenting with erotic activities that were per se very pleasurable and full of genuine love and respect, yet were not implicated in a sequential pattern that would eventually lead to a new monogamous relationship.

Back in Rome, good teachers were not difficult to find and delighted to get to work. I am especially grateful to Alberto, who was about twice my age and taught me how to get all of my body involved in the lovemaking. I met him at Veronica's, who had been a model for Guttuso, a very sensual Italian painter of the modernist generation— the warm aura of his gaze still lingering on her. She also searched for a mode of sexual play better than with her husband, Claudio, but had a hard time getting over the trauma of being raped by her uncle at age nine on a Sardinian country road. Veronica and I were true confidantes, and so the magic worked! Alberto was a retired Italian army colonel, with a trim body, a nice tan, and some gray hair. He had the somewhat formal manners typical of the military, but in intimate situations he would switch to a much more sanguine, spontaneous mode. He had a trailer in the parking lot of some military airport and from what I could tell, he was out of a long-term relationship that had turned sour, but had been good sex all the way. With him it was pure sex, but his techniques were perfect and the student was more than ready. Alberto helped me discover the eroticism of hands, feet, legs, shoulders, belly, and all other parts of the body that are often not considered especially erogenous. He would flip his tongue all over my body so that all of my skin would awake. He was very patient and always demonstrated first. He'd focus on my pleasure and did not expect much in return. When I flinched he would catch me right on so I stayed in the game. I learned that good male lovers learn to satisfy their female partners first, so that both partners can enjoy together later, and their next expression of sexual attention will be welcome. I found out that a man's control over his own erection, or at least his modesty and ability to make up for it in other ways, is an essential part of good male sexual education. If it were more widespread, wouldn't the world be a happier and more peaceful place? I was learning to be a good student to become a good teacher someday.

XXIII
Terrorism

In the fall of 1981, I regarded my enrollment in the UC Riverside master's program as a temporary journey. As an Italian girl whose relatives had moved to Rome from the Apennines and Naples, I had ancestral memories of trips to America made by people who never returned and had disappeared even from their loved ones' memories. They were the mostly illiterate peasants and unskilled laborers who formed the body of the mass exodus from the Southern Italian region of *Meridione* that took place between the unification of 1870 and the World War I years. In American popular culture they would be known as the likes of Leonardo DiCaprio's character in the movie *Titanic*. They had all of the rough charm, the illusions, and energy that made him feel prepared to leave everything behind and start over. But popular mythology presented them as persons who would disappear, or at least whose names and souls would change so radically that they would no longer remember the vocalic ending of their original last names, nor would they know which Southern hometown their family was from. Of the many songs in the Italian popular tradition, the one that most occurred to me in this period went, "Mama, gimme one hundred lira for to America I wanna go. Here's to you, here's to you, but to America no no no!" *"Mamma mia dammi cento lire che in America voglio andar, cento lire io te le do, ma in America no no no!"* As if to confirm the mother's dire prediction, the song went on, "When they came to the open sea the ship started to fall below, and the waves and the waves washed away that head of curls." *"Quando furono in mezzo al mare il bastimento s'inabissò, e i capelli ricciuti e belli l'acqua del mare se li portò."* There was a sense of doom in this song that made me feel as if a part of me would be dead forever once I left for the New World.

Even so, a part of me *was* dead already, and as years passed, I reflected on that decision as one that partly resulted from the strange developments of the cultural and political movements in which I participated. The student rebellions of the 1960s had been followed by major, countrywide strikes in factories and public transportation. From the *autunno caldo,* the hot autumn of 1969, that had seen students and workers united in reclaiming rights for the subordinated, things had taken a more violent turn, as the promoters of a strategy of terror engineered a series of massacres designed to take control of the nation's soul. Many Italians like me and you lived next to the epicenters of this kind of organized violence. We didn't know who the promoters were and what was their ultimate goal, but we felt the burden of the instability their actions created. The sequence started with Piazza Fontana in Milan, where thirteen passersby died from a bomb placed near a bank. In the years to follow, the escalation of terrorism was marked by a similar massacre on the *Italicus* train, and by the capture and murder of Prime Minister Moro, in 1978. It culminated in another massacre, at the Bologna Railway Station in 1980, where eighty-five people were killed. This may not seem like a lot to you today, but at that time the globe was a healthier place.

Terrorist organizations embraced various political ideologies. *Ordine nuovo,* or The New Order, claimed a Fascist legacy. Others were more Luddite and anarchistic in nature, including *Autonimia operaia,* Workers' Autonomy, and *Gruppi armati proletari,* or Proletarian Armed Bands. *Lotta continua,* or Continuing Struggle, was more student based and ideologically oriented. Many participants were in good faith, and ironically they were the ones to pay the highest price when the system was dismantled in the late 1980s. The most legendary terrorist organization was of course the *Brigate rosse,* or Red Brigades, which was often blamed for everything, especially abroad. But other organizations were often more noxious and capable of hiding their tracks. As you know, my friends and family were leftists and we shared a color symbolism with them, but we could not share their intent, because their vision seemed to be based on the idea that it was best to destroy the liberal capitalist state rather than to gradually transform it into something else. Like most prominent people in the left who did not share the ideology of terrorism, your grandpa Dario was in a delicate position. Was it more important to establish one's ideological distance from the Red Brigades, or to claim that their people were misled and probably sponsored by the CIA?

Grandpa's *Sinistra indipendente,* or Independent Left, was a way to answer that question indirectly. As a former vice minister who had refused to stick with his fellow cabinet members, he was unattached and free to establish the connections he wanted, both politically and ideologically. The independent group was a way to create a political space where progressives could gather and collaborate, regardless of their belief systems and ideologies. Formed under the auspices of the largest Communist Party on this side of the Iron Curtain, Dario's group helped the PCI establish its reputation as a champion of democratic pluralism which had cut the umbilical chord that attached it to Moscow. But his position was especially delicate, since, as the founder of a group that believed in the cooperation between democracy and socialism, his political career depended on the possibility that this collaboration develop in a peaceful way. His success was dependent on the willingness of both Christian Democracy and Communist Party to collaborate. In each party there were different currents. Hard liners on either side would rather stick to their own guns. But visionary, inclusive leaders such as Moro and PCI's Enrico Berlinguer wanted to negotiate a plan together, so as to stabilize the system and generate more prosperity for everyone. This pleased neither hard liners nor terrorists, who had already decided that worse was better and were intent in the *tanto peggio tanto meglio* massacre game.

The house on the hill where we lived with your father in 1978 was a few bus stops away from my old place, where Grandpa Dario and uncle Andrea still lived. It was really a slingshot from via Mario Fani, where Prime Minister Moro lived with his family when he was abducted. As you know, your grandpa was a pacifist who had nonetheless fought in World War II, first as an army regular, then as a partisan, as soon as the volunteer anti-Fascist liberation brigades were formed. He was to be the main proponent for the conscientious objection bill the Italian parliament signed into law in the 1970s. He was a heart patient, and I remember him, in the heyday of the Red Brigades, getting the special permission to bear arms required by the Italian state, based on his apprehension about possible terrorist threats directed at him. It turned out he had good reasons to be apprehensive, for years later interpretations of the Moro case suggest his fellow party members, the hardliners, were the ones who abandoned him to the Red Brigades. Your father and I used to drive our bumpy *cinquecento,* you perched on the backseat of this diminutive Fiat vehicle designed to weasel its way through Italy's narrow roads. In the months when Moro was a prisoner of the terrorist organization, the police used to block the road just before the last light, and for days on end we were stopped and manually searched on our way home.

Perhaps my departure to the New World was a way to evade a situation where I saw no future for you or me. I admired Grandpa Dario's fierce independence, and wondered if he was aware it would drive his children away. But the system was besieged by opposing forces which polarized tensions that resulted from Italy's strategic position with respect to the Iron Curtain. We were the first country to the West of that divisive wall. Thanks to superpower ideology, we grew up knowing nothing about our Eastern neighbors—their mysterious world wrapped in a cloud of biased information behind the Iron Curtain. Little did we know that while they lay dying in a stagnant economy, we were enduring the growing pains of a country in the process of coming into postmodernity from a largely premodern state. From a *paese di fuga*—a country of flight that people leave to seek their fortune somewhere else—your beloved Italy was transforming into a *paese ospite,* a host country that attracts immigrants in search of their dreams of fortune and happiness. The left had been intent in pursuing its strategy of negotiating with the government rather than opposing it. It was mired in the contradiction of being positioned as ideologically opposed to this multiculturalization process, while many of its members were learning to enjoy its benefits, even as they kept their distance from the newcomers in many ways. Would Italians of your generation behave more mercifully to their guest workers than the German, French, American, Argentinean, and Australian hosts had behaved to the destitute Italian immigrants of yore? I crossed the ocean with a university degree and acquired another in the process only to find out that, for all my education, I was but a speck in that migrant flow anyway.

Part Three:
Epilogue

XXIV
Sacred Bi Love

The antique armoire was opposite to the queen-size bed in the large bedroom, next to a marble lavatory. The sunlight came in through the narrow window with the smell of beech trees from the garden below, as the mountain breeze stirred up their branches. On top of the armoire stood a wooden object about four feet long. It looked like a double sledge, with two pairs of arched legs, to which two parallel boards had been nailed. The boards were about one foot apart, blackened from overheating like most of the object itself. I opened my eyes and looked at it. *"Il prete,"* I remembered. The building had been around for about three centuries, and in the old days, when central heating did not exist, a little before bedtime people used to place a *prete* between the sheets to warm their beds. I recalled its bulge under the quilt in Grandma's bed, like a person cuddled in sleep, head buried under the blankets from the cold. Equipped with a brazier full of incandescent embers, in about fifteen minutes the *prete* would do its job. Then it would be refilled from the fireplace and passed on to another bed. "How come people call this a *prete?*" I remembered asking grandmother many years earlier, curious that people would use the Italian word for priest for these quite effective bedwarmers.

Teresa left the answer to my imagination.

It is the summer of 2000, and the World Gay Pride Parade takes place in Rome as a gay jubilee. In June I go to Italy to decide what to

This story was previously published in *Plural Loves: Designs for Bi and Poly Living,* 2004, Harrington Park Press and *Journal of Bisexuality* 4(3/4):199-218 © 2004 by The Haworth Press, Inc.

do with my property in Fosca, two hours away. Touching a soil that belongs to me brings back my memories. The night I arrive I've nothing to eat at home and I go out. The village is very compact. One can walk anywhere and there's only one restaurant. Tonina, the owner, recognizes me, and comes up to my table. We remember the last time I was there about ten years earlier.

"Fosca is now more diverse. We have one black person," she says.
"Who is it?"
"Well, our parish priest from Mozambique. Didn't you know?"
"Oh, really! How long has he been around?"
"About a year. He speaks three languages, is very cultured, and people love him. He's nice, and he got us all involved in a council that helps him run the parish. I'm part of it, did you know? Besides, he's not like a typical priest. He doesn't wear a gown, he is social, he likes people, he's got many friends already. I'll introduce him to you. You'll see, he's so amiable."
"Sure, I'd love to meet him."

A couple of days later another female friend, Silvana, hands me a business card. It reads Reverend Jean-Luc Feleon, with phone number and cellular. Silvana is a cousin of Tonina, since in that village everybody is related.

"I told Jean-Luc all about you, that you're back in town after so long, that you live in America and speak many languages, that you've been all over the place. Jean-Luc wants to meet you," she says. "You can call him any time."

I don't do priests, and I'm not even a Catholic. But in this hometown people are so boring I'm thrilled that someone more interesting is around. The same weekend is patron saint's day, San Calisto. I'm told that Mass will be celebrated on the church's landing, for the old building has been condemned, typical of the area. I tell myself, *Gaia, you can check him out. You don't even have to get into the church. Just get yourself there before Mass is over.* And so I do. It is amazing.

On the steep mountain slope past the river and the narrow valley, medium-sized beech trees fill the landscape behind the minister's head. The soft pillow of his well-combed kinky hair forms a black aura around his face. The small medieval church is to his left, with its okra stones and cordoned entrance. The townspeople are gathered in the landing. Most of them are old, and I can recognize the way they are related from their facial traits. The women's faces look like so many saints' portraits, tight pink lips as in prayer, high.cheekbones turned red by the brisk mountain air, brown eyes and wavy hair turning gray. Their bodies are trim and sturdy, with bony limbs and bulky chests. The men's sunburned faces have deep creases and bristly facial hair. Their heavy potbellies protrude above their leaner legs.

There are only three or four main families in this village, and they've intermarried for so long that they all look alike. I'm a hybrid comparatively, since I'm only one-fourth from there. I can see the shape of my grandmother's thin nose on the faces of many women who are for sure her cousins or nieces or some other relation. I look at this group of people, all so provincial, so inbred. *A very shallow gene pool,* I think. And then I look at the altar, where their spiritual guide is celebrating the main ritual of their religion, turning bread into human flesh and then offering it to the faithful. The dark of his skin is translucent with deep purple and red. The embroidered garments are white, green, and gold. They look gorgeous against his colors. His hands are raised to receive the universal energy, and the white of his outstretched palms shines against the fine mountain air. The gown itself makes him look feminine, like a transvestite. He is very erotic in a natural way. As he speaks I notice his Italian is perfect, of the kind spoken only by educated foreigners. *He must be a good student,* I think to myself. I notice a lot of younger women go to communion these days. They must be excited; it's all so erotic. I feel a contraction in my vaginal walls. Then the singing starts, and the procession begins to flow. I follow with others as we chatter away.

I'd never been with a priest yet, but I remembered a movie about a gay priest I saw. I was surprised that seeing a priest as an erotic creature had made me uncomfortable, as if I was in denial of their sexuality. A couple of days later I see Jean-Luc on the low-level wall on the other side of the road from the small church where they have Mass on weekdays. It is dusk, and I am walking down the main street, where people socialize everyday. Of course I cannot miss him. He wears a civilian shirt in earth tones, and I notice the colors are very becoming to him. He is talking to Tonina, the restaurant owner, and Rina, another neighbor. They all look very happy and friendly. I am wearing shorts, which is still considered audacious in the area.

I walk toward them, and say to him, "I'm Gaia, the woman Silvana told you about, the one who lives in America."

He looks out and thinks for a moment. "Oh, Gaia, yes, the woman who speaks English and French, and just returned from America. I'm so glad to meet you, Gaia," and he puts out his hand. Well, we try out our French, then our Spanish. We tell each other a bit about our lives, where we'd lived, and why, and so on. The others feel a bit lost.

He says, "My brother is coming," and he points to a car up the road. We walk there, and I am introduced. "Here's another minister from Mozambique. His name is George, and he speaks English as well as Italian and French."

The three of us walk to the *casa parrocchiale,* the parish priest's premises. I look at the books in there, a computer, the office, something very advanced for a town like that. Jean-Luc shows me a book on spiritual trances in Mozambique, and explains it is the doctoral dissertation of one of his friends. Then George asks me what kind of food I prefer.

"Chinese."

"Let's go," he says, and we go out.

We take two cars, for George has to go on to Rome, while I am coming back to Fosca with Jean-Luc. I ride with George. He asks, "What kind of music do you prefer?"

"New Age."

"Really? But, would you mind explaining to me what is this New Age?"

"Of course! It's the movement that brought about a return to a more spontaneous spirituality. New Paganism is my favorite variety. The sacred is in the earth, and the main deity is feminine. She knows what we are doing to her, and is not happy. Those who understand this love and respect her. All things, animated and not, are sacred, and we, humans, are guests just like everybody else."

"Do you know anything about polyfidelity?"

I think, *What an interesting priest. I didn't know priests were aware of this stuff at all.*

"I've been a holistic health practitioner in North County San Diego, and that's where I've learned to get past monogamy and honor erotic and spiritual impulses in a more cosmic way. I was part of a polyamorous community and loved it for I could love more than one person at a time without cheating. And it's so erotic, with so many people in a love embrace, the energy multiplies, and everything feels so much better."

I am talking about these things with a Catholic priest, I think briefly as I hear myself continue. "I'm gay, and more specifically bisexual, and I've had these wonderful experiences in Southern California."

"But how do you transfer these things. How do you export them?"

"You don't. For people to feel comfortable with their erotic energy, there has to be a conducive environment, and that can only come gradually with a lot of education."

We eventually get to the Chinese restaurant, and there I am having dinner with two good-looking black priests in civilian clothes, talking about new age spirituality and other heresies. We all have a terrific time. It feels like family. I'm a foreigner in Italy, for when I go back I always feel so different from those who stayed.

On the way back it is dark. I have never been that close to a priest. I look at Jean-Luc, and notice he doesn't look like any African Americans or Africans I know. *He looks Italian,* I think to myself, *Italian in a way that I don't anymore. He looks sweet and sexy, and without intending it—at least, one cannot tell he is posing. He is seductive in a spontaneous way.* Sure enough we start talking about celibacy.

"I am aware that the topic is now being debated within the Church," I observe. "Clearly, there is a lack of callings; the church will need to change its rules if it wants to have any priests at all."

He agrees. "I have five parishes. It's a lot of work. Five villages, all under the jurisdiction of only one priest. Lots of Masses to celebrate, funerals, baptisms, communions, everything else. And imagine, I'm a graduate student. This is supposed to be a part-time job. I don't even have time to think about my graduate work."

He takes off his eyeglasses for a moment and I can see the thick rim of his lashes around his eyeballs. It looks as if he has some permanent makeup on!

"Not many Italians want to be priests anymore," he continues. "Working on Sundays, never being off, no early retirement, no marriage."

"There used to be a time when talented boys from indigent families were recruited into seminary," I reply. "That way they could get an education instead of tending goats. Then some stayed in the church, some got out and became teachers and so on. I know people who've done that. That option was never available to women though, did you know?"

I turn my face and notice his heart-shaped lips, of a light-brown color fading into pink. A hearty smile lightens their pink spot. I imagine how they would feel on mine, both above and below.

"But what do you think?" he says. "Do you expect a priest to be celibate to respect him, to think he is a good priest?"

I am a bit surprised by the question. What do I think? "Well," I say, "I never went to church because my parents were atheists. I'm not a Catholic, and priests never had charisma for me. I didn't care whether or not they were celibate. But lately I've surprised myself. I read the memoir of a woman who had a relationship with a priest for thirty years, and even had three children by him. It was so passionate, inspiring. The way she described their relationship was so exciting, erotic. I consider myself a very liberated person, and yet, this was new to me. I thought to myself, *Gaia, are you being squeamish or curious?* I'm still not sure, but, tell me, have I answered your question?"

He smiles and says, *"Si, certo.* Yes you have, dear; you sure have!"

"Now I have a question," I say. "I get the feeling your sexual desires are very strong. How do you feel about them? Are you comfortable? Where do you stand?"

He looks into the night as the curved road keeps climbing the mountain slope. The off-white collar of his shirt brushes against his ebony jaw. "The celibacy of priests is an issue of ecclesiastic right, not of divine right. It was decided by humans, not by God. I do not see this law as necessary."

The answer surprises me in its clarity and directness. It certainly deserves an A.

At night I keep tossing and turning in bed. I have wet dreams and his body feels almost as real as flesh under the blankets. I have a vision of his heart-shaped lips and black-rimmed eyes on my pillow. I wake up at 9 a.m. and call him.

"It's so nice to hear your voice. Did you sleep well?"

"I had dreams of you, as if you were here."

"I can visit you."

"When?"

"This morning?"

"Okay. What time?"

"In an hour or so."

"Great! See you then."

He comes to my place and I give him a tour of the house. Then we sit on the sofa, and we kiss. He wears a gray suit and a white shirt. The flat stripe between the two flaps of his collar marks him as clergy. His lips are sweet like honey. He gets up and takes the collar off. It makes me horny. We sit down again. He is embarrassed. I think, *Maybe he hasn't been with a white woman yet. Maybe he is afraid I will blab.*

"I am divorced," I explain. "I'm free and I don't want to marry." He seems relieved.

"What kind of sex have you had before?" I ask.

He is a bit shy, reluctant. "It's been about a year, with a gal I met in the library doing research."

"If we like each other and respect each other, and know what we want, we can have a *storia*." *Storia* is the Italian word for a love affair, except that it doesn't have its negative connotations. Like a fling, but deeper.

"Do you think we could really do that?"

"I'm the right person. We're neighbors, but I'm not really one of your parishioners, for I'm not a Catholic and I'm on vacation." We kiss some more and touch all over. We're half undressed and I say, "Let's go to the bedroom. It's better there."

We rush, our pants half down. I explain we only have a half hour to go. We get undressed and into bed. He looks at my body, elongated and dainty, with a soft, padded belly and round breasts. The ash gold of my skin glows against his translucent ebony. He is a fine lover, with a well-functioning dick and much control. But I realize I'm going to have to give him some safer-sex lessons. *Good for you, Gaia,* I think to myself.

"I am a safer-sex educator," I explain. "I use condoms, and you must wear one or I will get pregnant." He stops and lets me lubricate his dick and slide the condom on. I'm proud of exercising my educational skills. We finish off rather quickly, but the chemistry is so good we promise to do this again soon, with more time on our hands.

Next time we get together is for dinner at his home. His brother is back. We speak English, for George and I prefer it. He tags along. *A bit weak in this language,* I notice. For some reason we get back on the polyamory conversations.

"Polyamorous people practice safer sex with all partners except one, their primary. My partner Emily and I, for example, had other lovers, but we exchanged fluids only between ourselves." Before I know it, I feel my face blush up to my earlobes. *I've given myself away,* I think. *It's not the fear of losing him, but the shame for not telling him before.* I'm not sure they notice my embarrassment, and I keep myself going. After dinner his brother goes home, and here I am, in the parish priest's home, fornicating on the sofa. We eventually move to the bed, which is upstairs, very small.

"I'm queer, bisexual. Your brother already knew. I am sorry for not telling earlier." I whisper as we lie down. No response.

We lie down chest against chest. He has cute nipples with no chest hair. I hold one between my fingers. My nipples are perky and he holds one as well. It's like magic. Erotic ecstasy. And we need to do absolutely nothing to keep it going. The energy flows between the aroused nipples and the fingers that hold them. We're on a tantric plateau, and we stay there till about 1 a.m. We smile and our lips are turgid with joy, our bodies alive and beautiful with erotic energy. We check that the street is clear. I rush out as quietly as possible, and slip myself inside my home. I have the sweetest dreams. I feel elated and happy.

We plan our next meeting as a road trip. The village is small, and I'm sure Tonina noticed that the evening we met, the three of us went to a Chinese restaurant out of town instead of hers. I'm still kind of worried about that, thinking of ways to make it up to her. I'm walking uphill on a paved mountain road towards a nearby village, and he's supposed to pick me up. We drive to a sanctuary, in the nearby town of Cascia. We visit the church. I realize what this means to him. I feel the sacred energy despite Catholicism. More talking.

"I've thought of leaving the ministry many times, marrying, having babies." I see the longing in his eyes.

In a way, as long as he is in Italy, he is condemned to being a priest bound to his celibacy vows. He is an *extracomunitario,* namely not a citizen of the European Union. If he left the church he would lose his right to work. If he were not a priest, he'd be just one in a million marginalized people of color who often resort to illegal activities to make ends meet in the rich Italian economy of today. I surprise myself thinking that his dignity depends on the Catholic Church, which brought multiculturalism to Fosca's deep province. *His brother and he are probably the most cultured and well-read persons in the area. Italy is multiculturalizing at a fast pace, but are Italians ready for what that really means, are they prepared to have these new people protected and integrated?* I remember myself as a graduate student in Southern California, many, many years earlier, looking forward to proving myself in what I thought was a better world. Wanting, at the same time, to become part of it and to learn its secrets and take them back home. *Of course, he could leave the church if I married him,* I think to myself. *But then the magic between us would be lost.*

We meander through the curvy road half way up on the mountain slope. I feel grateful for this encounter, this joy. We stop for dinner at a local *trattoria.* He has *primo e secondo*, a first and a second course. I don't. A succulent plate of spaghetti with *Amatriciana* sauce lies before him. He eats it with gusto, properly rolling the noodles on his fork. *He is more Italian than I am,* I think to myself. I quit doing the sequence of double entrees typical of Italian meals a long time ago.

He spends the evening at my place. This time we make love in a more artistic way. I explain that I like to do it well. We have plenty of time, and my bedroom is large and comfortable. I play Loreena

McKennitt on the stereo. I turn the electric heater on. I burn some incense. Under the pillow, I prepare my safer-sex toys. A lubricant called For-Play, a nice medium-size vibrator, a large ostrich feather, a pair of Chinese balls. He takes off his glasses, and I notice his rimmed eyes again. He is puzzled about my protests of being gay.

"What do women do together?" he asks.

"Huh," I say. "So you're curious, ha?" He looks at me. "Well, do you want me to show you how you can please a woman if you are a woman yourself?"

"I do," he says. "I've heard about these things, these toys that women use. Do you have them?"

"I do."

"Really?" He is excited. "Can I see them?"

"Of course," I say, and I start fumbling around under the pillow. I unwrap the dildo and hold it out. "See, it's just like a penis, except it always works." I turn it on and move it nearer his face. "It's got a nice buzz, feel that?" He stays interested. "But you've got to know what to do with it," I continue. "Do you know how women come, how they feel pleasure?"

"Well, I know some," he says. "I'm sure there's a lot more. Explain!"

"I'll give you the map to a woman's pleasure," I say as I spread my legs. I feel a bit like Annie Sprinkle, and tell myself that I'm doing the day's good work. I point to the entrance of my vagina, "This is the pleasure site you used yesterday," I explain. "It's wonderful, but it's not the only one a woman has. You must be aware of the others as well. There is the clit, and the anus, which you have also." I move my fingers up and show my small labia and the clitoris inside. "A woman feels intense pleasure when she receives clitoral stimulation," I explain. "Can you see that little button between the small labia?" He comes closer and looks more carefully. "Well, my female lover used to spend hours holding it between her lips and pressing it with her tongue."

He looks perplexed. *He probably got more than he bargained for,* I reflect. I take the dildo in my hands and turn it on. I press it against my clit. "That's how you use this on a woman's genitals," I demonstrate.

"Yesterday, when you penetrated me, I had a vaginal orgasm," I continue, "but you did not stimulate my clit. You can give me a clitoral orgasm with this, or with your fingers. You need to stimulate the entire area, inside the vagina, near the entrance, around the labia, and finally on the clit. The clit is a very delicate object. If properly stimulated, it swells up like a small penis, if not, it hurts." I turn the dildo off.

"Can I put my fingers inside you?" he asks.

"Of course." I show him how to make a small dildo with his three fingers, and guide him inside. My walls tighten up. He looks at me. "See, you're making love to me like a woman now."

He takes the dildo in his hand and turns it on. He starts to play with it as he looks at my genitals. It feels wonderful. I remember the first love lessons I gave Stephane when he was in my Italian course. It started like a game, and then I fell in love. *It might happen again,* I think to myself, realizing how deeply, for me, learning and eroticism are related. *I must be a good teacher,* I reflect, as Jean-Luc is intensely absorbed in his playing with my genitals. *I love this erotic pedagogy. If only I could teach this to my college students as well!*

He uses the dildo very well, pointing its tip between my clit and the entrance to my vagina. After a while I feel a liquid flowing between my legs, it comes out of the area he is stimulating, it is warm and its ejection gives me an intense pleasure. I am not entirely sure what is happening, though. I touch his hand and gently push it away. I turn around and smell the area of the sheet under my legs. I am afraid I've been incontinent! But no, the liquid has no smell. It occurs to me that I have probably just experienced female ejaculation. I smile at him. He is confused.

"You made me ejaculate! Did you know that nobody has ever done that before? I have never even been able to make a woman ejaculate myself." I point to the wet sheets, and put his fingers on them. "Can you feel that?"

"Yes, I can."

"Well, that's a liquid that came out of my genitals. I've never seen it before. I've only heard about it from my bi friends, and I've seen it in soft porn." I am thinking of Annie Sprinkle's *Sluts and Goddesses*.

"This is female ejaculation," I repeat. "I can't believe you've done that." I start to doubt the sincerity of his naïveté. "Are you sure you're as new to this as you say?"

He lowers his eyes and there is surprise on his face. Then he looks at me and says, "Gaia, is something wrong? I'm doing as you tell me."

"No, I was just thinking that you beat all of my other lovers in just one lesson. I thought you might have done these things before and pretended you were just learning them."

He doesn't answer.

"Forgive me," I say. "It doesn't really matter."

We resume the play, with more warm ejaculations. Eventually, my clitoral orgasm comes. He keeps watching the results of his work as in an ecstasy. I point to how my anal orifice is now softer and more open. "It's connected to the clit," I explain.

"Can we use it?" he asks.

"Let's leave that for our next lesson," I suggest. Then I show him how to put a condom on, and he penetrates me. I notice the usual control. His dick is slender and a bit curved, its veins pulsating under the thin skin. I look at his shape lying down on the bed, the translucent ebony of his body is smooth like jungle dew and emanates the most aphrodisiac smells. I get on top and ride him until I come, the kundalini energy rising from my sacrum to the back of my head. Then we turn around and he comes softly, whispering my name. We lie down and he says, "Tonight was better. I saw you come. It was great."

"That's part of having sex that's queer, artsy, a bit gay, if you want. You and your partner take turns. You get to watch the other person and live their pleasure. Then they do the same. Isn't that better than the missionary position?"

"What's the missionary position?" he asks.

"What do you mean? Don't you know?"

"I sure don't."

He has proven himself such a great lover that I am embarrassed to explain. "Missionary," I say. "It's called missionary position because Christian missionaries used to teach it to the savages in former colonies as the only acceptable way to make love." The irony of the situation requires no further comment. *What a great student,* I tell myself. *He surpassed the teacher on his first lesson.*

I speak a bit about the Fosca I knew from my memories and my family's. "Most people didn't have great sex in this town," I explain, "and that was the fault of the clergy and how they had always scared them that pleasure was bad. The missionary position was very widespread! The climate too, so cold in the winter that people had to always wear long underwear, even in bed. No divorcees, no single people past twenty-five or so, and buildings so packed together that you can hear your neighbors breathe. When push comes to shove," I keep going, "the parish priest was the only wild card in the village, no wonder he was supposed to hop from bed to bed." I point to the *prete* on top of the armoire. "He was like one of those traditional bedwarmers full of incandescent embers. It was part of his pastoral mission, in a way," I tease him.

He smiles with his eyes lowered, the pink of his lips lucent with serene joy. "Now that I taught you all these wonderful tricks to give women pleasure, you can be generous. There is at least one beautiful and sensual woman in this town who is, I believe, a good lover, and her bed is cold. Silvana and her late husband Mario were always good lovers, both of them butchers by trade, somewhat familiar with flesh. But now Silvana is alone. I wonder if she's ever been with a woman, even in her imagination. But I won't be here to find out, and you can certainly warm up her bed." He doesn't pick up on this polyamorous note.

As we lie down, he looks at my belly, and touches it with his hands.

"This belly," he says.

"What?"

"Well, you told me I need to use condoms because you have your periods, right?"

"Uh-huh," I say.

"I thought you might have lost it already. That you were menopausal. Aren't you over forty?"

"Yes, I am, but my period is actually very regular, which it wasn't before. Maybe it's because I'm healthier, vegetarian and so on."

"You could bake me a couple of kids in that belly," he ventures.

"A couple of kids? I'm way past reproductive age. I just turned forty-five!"

"I don't have any kids."

"You can't," I reply. "It's the life you've chosen."

He looks serious, like the person who feels he is treated unfairly because he does not really belong. "Priests don't have a retirement plan, they often die poor and forgotten. If at least they had children, they could be taken care of," he says. "In Mozambique, Catholic priests from abroad have a couple of women they call wives, and they have children with them. When they retire, they have a place to go."

"Really?"

"Yes."

"But I'm not sure a minister can be also a good parent. Your pastoral mission is loving all people in exactly the same way. How could you give your children the special love they need, and love unconditionally all the children in the world as well?"

He does not answer, and I think he probably believes himself capable of that kind of love. *Does he know that if the Vatican was not as misogynist as a medieval monastery, he probably wouldn't even be here?* I realize how ambitious he is. Coming all the way from Mozambique to the center of the institution he wants to be part of. It occurs to me that, even though I despise the Catholic universities of Rome, for people in the ecclesiastic career, these schools are the top of tops. A bit like Yale for academics in the United States. I imagine raising his child in Fosca, where everybody would know who his father is. People would stare at him, "the priest's child," they'd giggle. In my grandmother's time, there were two ways to call someone a bastard, and one was *"figlio del prete."*

"So, you want to have a child, right?" I say. "What about women who don't even get to be priests at all?"

"Well, I never said women shouldn't be priests. I just want to have a child from you, a child like you."

In my sleep I feel the force of a debt pound against my chest. I call Jean-Luc the next morning. "Can I please see you?" I say, "I have to tell you something important. It is part of your pastoral mission to hear it."

"Come over. I'm home."

I walk to his place, he opens the door, and we go into the study. We sit in front of each other and I take his hands into mine. I look at him and say, "You've given me two wonderful gifts, and I want you to know that I am immensely grateful." I pause for breath. "One is that you made me ejaculate, and now I know it's possible and I can give that gift to another person. The other is that you asked to have a child with me. It's a great honor that you gave me, and I have no words to thank you."

"Does this mean we can have a baby then?" he asks.

"No, but it means that I want to thank you for asking me." I put my arm next to his. The sunlight from the window makes our skins glow. "He or she would have a wonderful color," I say, "and would be a wonderful child. Thank you!"

At night Jean-Luc comes for his second lesson. Dinner is ready. As we eat he watches all the antique furniture, the objects, the memories of my whole family that I have there. I show him the chiaroscuro pencil drawing I made of Michelangelo's *Pietà* when I was about twelve. It is framed and hangs from the dining room wall.

"You guys are not such atheists, then," he observes.

"Well, my grandparents were not. It started with my parents. I think my father's atheism is just a reaction to the tyranny of the Catholic Church. In Italy, there is only one religion. As I got to California, I realized there were many, and they all coexisted. I remember one day wondering, 'Buddha looks Asian, Allah looks Middle Eastern, and Jesus looks white. What a coincidence,' I reflect. 'They're all men. How come their religions claim men were made in God's image? To me it looks like it was the reverse.' That's how I started to get past atheism and reach out for a belief system I could call my own."

"How do you feel now about Catholicism?"

"To me, it's a primitive religion," I observe. "It's monotheistic; it's male oriented, and I mean both in a negative way. I want a world with many deities, and one in which the divine principle is feminine; it's in the earth."

"Why don't you come to Mass sometime? You might feel a spiritual connection even though it's not your belief system, you know?"

"Well, to be honest with you, this is the only town where I ever like to go, because it's so simple and genuine. I'll come if you are sure to understand that for me Mass is nothing but a cannibalistic ritual performed by a transvestite."

He lowers his eyes, and smiles peacefully. "I get the cannibalism, but the transvestite?"

"Well, don't you celebrate it in a colorful gown?"

"Oh, okay," he says, and his lips open showing more of the pink inside. "Then I'll be waiting for you."

I know that the neighbors are gossiping already. In this town there's no way to keep people from finding out what's going on. I feel, "Well, if I show up those bigoted old ladies will believe he has converted me. That will be a success for him. I owe him that much!" So I show up on Sunday at twelve. It is a great moment. The church is full of men and women of all ages, children and families. He has girls and boys recite some of the prayers. He preaches well, and makes the whole church come alive with his words. I notice he mentions Christ's energetic body, his powerful aura, and the healing energy that it emanated. The sacredness of the space comes across to me very strong.

That evening we meet again, this time to make love. "I want to have anal sex with you," I explain, "for it's the strongest orgasm I can have. But it takes me a lot of excitement to get there and really enjoy it. If I'm not ready it's very painful." I'm on all fours, my pussy juicy and swollen with anticipation. I show him how to arouse me and get the anus to open. I lead his hand to the hood and clit. He moves it up and down the labia, spreading the wet juice all the way to the anus. Now the sphincter is opening and his turgid cock slides in like into a glove. I feel orgasmic vibrations throughout the area, the kundalini energy going up through the spine to the back of my head. I am happy, for once, to let him come without a condom, since I don't really believe in HIV infection, and practice safer sex for protection against other STDs and pregnancy.

"I want you to feel what I felt, and will penetrate you with a toy," I explain when we're expended. Then I proceed to do just that. He lies down on his belly, and I notice the light on his translucent shoulders, his butt a bit perky, tightened up as if he was afraid of a nurse's shot. I put my finger on his anus, which feels very closed. I realize my dildo is too large, and use my finger instead. I get almost all of it in there. It is the first time for me also. "What do you feel?" I ask.

"It's painful," he says, as the pink of his lips shows. "It's the first time."

He is willing to stay in the game, I think, as I keep going until he begins to feel the pleasure. I move my finger up and down his ass. I love to see a man's body subject itself to being penetrated. There is a vulnerability that cannot come across in any other way. I feel the flesh inside him quiver around my finger, and remember the first time I penetrated a woman in a similar way. I look at his face pressed against the sheets, his mind feeling his body alive in a new way. I stop as I feel he got a taste of the forbidden pleasure and will want to get more.

"Can I stay for the night?" he asks.

"I prefer to sleep alone."

"Let's meet tomorrow and drive to George's home," he says as he puts his clothes on.

We meet as usual, on the road well outside the town. I have been walking for about an hour under the midday sun, and am kind of tired and worried.

"I always have lots of people to answer and talk to after Mass," he says as I get in the car. "Besides, I did not want to rush out and create suspicion." We eat at George's, and I cannot help but notice that his place looks messy, as if he does not have his life in order. *I'm sure that adjusting to the Central Apennines is difficult when you come from Boston,* I think to myself. We leave soon after lunch, on my suggestion, and stop the car in a nearby meadow to neck in the bushes. It is my idea, and I realize that he is uncomfortable because we have no viper antidote. I have forgotten, since there are no vipers in North America! We get back to the car. The air is brisk, and the large valley is filled up with the waters of an artificial lake. The hills and plateaus around are covered with green pastures. As we come to the main road, I notice he feels drowsy at the wheel.

"Can I take it?

"Please do. I'm sleepy. It's nap time for me, you know."

I think, *How Italian!*

We get to Fosca, and he goes to bed. He visits again later, and I show him pictures of my family, myself as a kid, my brother, cousins, parents. He is very curious. "You know so much about this town," he says. "You make me see it in a whole different way."

"I want to share all I know with you, so you can use it to your advantage and have an easier time doing your job. I want you to be successful, for I think you are a great blessing here."

"But what about us? Are we going to see each other again?"

"You know, my girlfriend Emily stayed in Southern California when I moved to Puerto Rico. Since then I really haven't had a partner. I love to be single, and don't know what will make me change my mind yet. I've moved so many times, I'm almost afraid to commit to a relationship, since that often means committing to a place as well. I'm an immigrant like you, you know? But this place is different. You're lucky. Every time I come I think I'll sell, then when I see the light come through the window as I've seen it since I can remember, I think if I sold this place I'd be lost. I want to keep it instead. So, if you're here when I come back, we will see each other again, yes. This place is a *punto fermo,* a pivotal point, and that's where I met you. Of course, you might be gone next time, you might get a better parish, and you should take it. But if you don't . . ."

"A pivotal point," he repeats. "I have one at home as well. I'm having a house built on a property in Mozambique, near my relatives, and that will be my *punto fermo* some day. Thanks for reminding me that it's important, that it matters to you as well. The world spins around so fast, and things change, and when you are abroad you always feel expendable, as if there was no firm ground under your feet. I know I wanted to get away, and I'm happy, but sometimes I feel lost, because, like you, I feel the whole world spins without a *punto fermo.* But now that you tell me that for you it is important, I'll be sure to create one for myself as well."

"I wish you the best of luck," I say, thinking that ironically when it's time for me to return to my pivotal point, when I retire that is, it might be time for him to go home.

The next day he drives me to a nearby town to go to the bank. We are entering a tunnel when he says, "But this being gay, this being queer, is it so necessary? I'm sure one needs to feel compassion for gays, understand them, but wouldn't it be best to help them change?"

"Change?" I answer. "Meaning what?"

"Well, change their ways, move on to the right direction."

I say no word.

"Being gay can't be natural, can it? Besides gays are always made fun of. Why be gay if you don't have to?" His tone is getting pressing, which is a typical way for Italians to debate issues about which they feel very strongly.

"Sleeping with you doesn't make me straight. I'm the one who decides what I am."

"But it doesn't seem right," he insists, somewhat mocking.

"I don't like that tone," I say. "These are not things to make fun of."

"Is that what I'm doing?" he teases.

"I'm not Italian! I'm not Italian!" I yell. "You can't discuss things with me this way. . . . I am speaking Italian with you and it might sound natural to you, but I'm not all that fluent and comfortable, and I don't like to discuss things at a fast pace."

A long silence follows. Then, "I didn't mean to offend you," he says, "I'm sorry."

"I don't like the way things are discussed in this culture. It's irrational and it makes people upset. That's the reason why everybody has heart failure. If you want to know more about what being bisexual means to me, you can ask me gently, and I'll be happy to tell you."

He has his sweet smile on his face. He is going to tease me for "not being Italian" for quite some time, but he gets my point. "Okay," he says, "tell me all about being bisexual."

"To you bis might seem just freaks, extravagant types who are fixated with some kind of kinky sex. But if you knew gay cultures from the inside, you would know that to each other gay people are like family. Queer people often don't have a family, because we've been repudiated. Our relatives live thousands of miles away, and they don't want to hear about us for they are ashamed. So queers form communities that are a bit like families. When I was in Southern California I barely had any contact with my relatives. They didn't understand why I was there, and wanted to manipulate me into being 'normal.' The bisexual community of San Diego was my family then. And they were a wonderful family I love very intensely to this day. Bis are more open than gay men or lesbians, for they choose not to choose between women and men. You're an immigrant, you should know about most of this stuff already. Immigrant communities are somewhat like gay communities. We help each other, we understand each other, we speak the same language. Don't you have friends from Mozambique here in Italy?"

"Of course," he answers.

"Don't they feel a bit like family to you?"

"They do," he says. "I had my niece come here to study in Rome, and now she's like my local family. My brother is my neighbor as well. We speak our native language, and we cook Mozambican food as well. Honestly, I don't want to spend a lot of my time with them, but I'm sure glad they're around. I hadn't thought about gays that way. Thank you!"

He never objects to my being bi after that, which is not quite true of my atheist relatives. *Now I do have evidence that atheists can be more bigoted than priests,* I reflect.

"Remember I taught you to love me like a woman, and that a man's orgasm must always be last?"

"I do," he says.

"Well, these are things I learned from my queer friends, so now you are indebted to them. You're part of our community as well, as a student of love and erotic energy!"

The next day I get a call from my dad's girlfriend, Beatrice. "Your father is alone in Rome. Would you go and look after him?"

"I'm having terrific sex with an African priest I found in Fosca."

"I believe you! But still," she says. "Here's Dad."

"Gaia, how are you?" my dad says. "I really don't need any help."

"I'll be back in two days, and I'll introduce you to the new parish priest of your hometown. He's very black, from Mozambique."

By this time Dario is retired from politics and is an activist in the peace movement. He is a *terzomondista* as they call them in Italy, one who believes that if poor countries were allowed to do better, we would all be better off. After I came out to him on the occasion of Andrea's wedding, he has been my friend.

Jean-Luc is supposed to drive me to Rome. The day before we leave is feverish. Getting things ready, scheduling.

"What should I wear?" Jean-Luc asks me, tentative.

"Dress normal, not as if you are going to meet your future father-in-law, but not as a priest either!"

In the car we talk about the town's gossips, how to take care of them, and how to take control.

"Aren't you afraid someone will tell the bishop you have a lover?" I ask.

"What can the bishop do?" he replies. "You know, after Mass the other day the women in the council asked me about you. It was Tonina and Rina. They advised me, they said, to be careful, that I had been seen visiting you, and some people were gossiping. But the thing is, they're the ones who saw me and gossiped!"

"I know," I say. "They must be envious. How did you respond?"

"It wasn't very difficult," he says. "I've been in that position already. I said, 'But don't you see how lucky you are to have a towns-person so worldly, so educated? She knows more than all of you put together, and look what nasty rumors you are spreading about her!'"

"Is that what you said?" I ask. I cannot believe his chutzpah. He's so shameless . . . *A good match to you, Gaia,* I reflect. *He might get harassed a lot when he does not wear his clerical collar,* I imagine. Maybe that's how he learned about dildos and vibrators in confession—some cute girl describing her sins in minutest details to see how he'd respond.

When we get to my dad's neighborhood I see him lost, afraid. Mostly retired people live there, and they do not see many *extra-comunitari,* except for those who do housecleaning and care of the elderly. We have to wait in the courtyard for my father is late. We both miss the brisk mountain air. Finally my dad arrives and looks deceptively healthy. He is very friendly and welcomes Jean-Luc.

"I learned my Latin and math from one of your predecessors," my dad says as we sit to dinner. "When I grew up in Fosca, the priest was the most knowledgeable person."

In the kitchen I'm near the stove and cook some sausage. For once I play good girl. I think maybe Dad imagines we're lovers, and is happy, for he can see this guy is not a girl. It's a bit deceptive, of course, but I forgive myself. I hear them talk full of joy and energy. They disagree, but I know my dad loves to talk to ministers who have a sincere faith, and try to convert them to atheism. For the first time in my life, and I am forty-five years old, I feel comfortable with a lover in the same room with me and my dad. *If it had only started earlier,* I reflect, *we could have been a happy family.*

A few days later I call Jean-Luc from a public phone in Rome. I have just returned from the largest ever gay pride parade in Rome, on July 8, 2000. More than 200,000 people came. The demonstration was intended as a gay jubilee, affirming the presence of gay Catholics around the world, and the strength of gay communities within Catholic cultures.

"The World Gay Pride Parade was a big success," I say on the phone. "All the papers gave it rave reviews, the news as well."

"I know," he says, "I followed. A major part of myself is invested in this issue now because I love you." I could not have been a happier person.

That week I call him a few times for I am worried. Is the gossip going to spread? Is he going to be transferred away?

"Don't worry," he says. "The church council women asked me more questions, and this time I put them even better in their place."

"What did you say?" I ask.

"Well, I told them that happy people who aspire to being blessed with serene grace live their lives joyfully, and have no business meddling with the town's gossips."

I cannot believe my ears. *There is something new pagan in his philosophy,* I muse to myself. *Why have I always thought that only dumb people enter the clergy?*

The following week I invite Jean-Luc to visit me in Rome. We rent an apartment from an ecotourist organization. It is next to the clinic where my mother Delia died of cancer more than thirty years ago. When we drive up to it, I recognize the place and my blood chills in my veins. It is ominous. *Am I here to learn something or what?* I feel the healing energy of being near a person with a strong spirituality, even though it is based on a belief system I cannot share. We get inside. The apartment is really nice and fully equipped. The bedroom is large, with a queen-size bed in the center, and a twin bed on one side. Ideal for me, since I like to sleep in my own bed. We lie down and start to kiss. He knows he owes me one from the time before, when he forgot to come last and left my clit half turned on. He starts to play with it with his fingers while he looks at my face. The rose becomes all juicy and opened, it makes me think of a Host, slippery and wet when it enters your mouth and the saliva moistens it.

I ask him, "Do you like it?"

"Yes," and the rim around his eyes glows. He adds, ironic, "Isn't this saving you from being gay?"

The pleasure of feeling his body next to mine, and feeling him feel my pleasure, fills me with overwhelming joy.

"Salvami, allora, salvami," I whisper. "Go ahead and save me then."

XXV
Postepilogue

Sara graduated from college with a *laurea* in psychiatric and psychosocial rehabilitation from the *Università Cattolica* in Rome. Gaia went back to academe and made tenure at the University of Puerto Rico, Mayagüez. Her erotic and holistic wisdom have entered academic discourse with her, as the cultural energy of the Caribbean gradually entered her space. Dario passed away just a few months before September 11 and did not see the disfigured world of today. His bilingual book of poetry, *A Lake for the Heart/Il Lago del Cuore* has appeared in the United States for his daughter's translation. Jean-Luc continues to be a priest in Fosca. Sara met Maurizio and together they gave birth to Alessio. She is becoming a specialist in Montessorian education.

ABOUT THE AUTHOR

Serena Anderlini-D'Onofrio, PhD, recently guest edited two issues of the *Journal of Bisexuality* that were also published in book form: *Women and Bisexuality: A Global Perspective* and *Plural Loves: Designs for Bi and Poly Living* (both from Haworth). Her current work focuses on human ecology, emotional sustainability, and erotic expression. She earned her PhD at the University of California, Riverside, and is Professor in the Humanities at the University of Puerto Rico, Mayaguez. She has been the recipient of a grant from the Harry Ransom Humanities Research Center at the University of Texas, Austin, and has thrice been the recipient of a Seed-Money Grant from the University of Puerto Rico.

Dr. Anderlini-D'Onofrio's first book *The "Weak" Subject: On Modernity, Eros, and Women's Playwriting* is a comparative study of women's authorship in modern theater. In the past twenty years, her articles have appeared in numerous journals, including *Atenea; Carte Italiane; Diacritics; DisClosure; Feminist Issues; Italian Culture; Journal of Dramatic Criticism & Theory; Journal of Gender Studies; Leggere Donna; Literature, Consciousness, and the Arts, Nebula, Theater; VIA: Voices in Italian Americana; Women and Language; Women's Studies International Forum; Zengers;* and *Z Magazine.* She has also contributed to various edited works, including *Feminine Feminists: Cultural Practices in Italy, Natalia Gonzburg: A Voice of the Twentieth Century,* and *Franca Fame: A Woman Onstage.* She is the co-translator of *In Spite of Plato,* a book of feminist theory by Italian philosopher Adriana Cavarero.

Dr. Anderlini-D'Onofrio is now at work on a book on the politics of love and the world's future, and on a number of other works. Her first book has been translated into Italian and her English translation of Luigi Anderlini's poetry collection, *A Lake for the Heart,* is forthcoming.

Order a copy of this book with this form or online at:
http://www.haworthpress.com/store/product.asp?sku=5526

EROS
A Journey of Multiple Loves

_____in hardbound at $29.95 (ISBN-13: 978-1-56023-571-2; ISBN-10: 1-56023-571-3)

_____in softbound at $19.95 (ISBN-13: 978-1-56023-572-9; ISBN-10: 1-56023-572-1)

240 pages

Or order online and use special offer code HEC25 in the shopping cart.

COST OF BOOKS_____

POSTAGE & HANDLING_____
(US: $4.00 for first book & $1.50
for each additional book)
(Outside US: $5.00 for first book
& $2.00 for each additional book)

SUBTOTAL_____

IN CANADA: ADD 6% GST_____

STATE TAX_____
(NJ, NY, OH, MN, CA, IL, IN, PA, & SD
residents, *add appropriate local sales tax)*

FINAL TOTAL_____
(If paying in Canadian funds,
convert using the current
exchange rate, UNESCO
coupons welcome)

☐ **BILL ME LATER:** (Bill-me option is good on
   US/Canada/Mexico orders only; not good to
   jobbers, wholesalers, or subscription agencies.)
☐ Check here if billing address is different from
   shipping address and attach purchase order and
   billing address information.

Signature_____

☐ **PAYMENT ENCLOSED: $**_____

☐ **PLEASE CHARGE TO MY CREDIT CARD.**

☐ Visa ☐ MasterCard ☐ AmEx ☐ Discover
☐ Diner's Club ☐ Eurocard ☐ JCB

Account # _____

Exp. Date_____

Signature_____

Prices in US dollars and subject to change without notice.

NAME_____

INSTITUTION_____

ADDRESS_____

CITY_____

STATE/ZIP_____

COUNTRY_____ COUNTY (NY residents only)_____

TEL_____ FAX_____

E-MAIL_____

May we use your e-mail address for confirmations and other types of information? ☐ Yes ☐ No
We appreciate receiving your e-mail address and fax number. Haworth would like to e-mail or fax special
discount offers to you, as a preferred customer. **We will never share, rent, or exchange your e-mail address
or fax number.** We regard such actions as an invasion of your privacy.

Order From Your Local Bookstore or Directly From
The Haworth Press, Inc.
10 Alice Street, Binghamton, New York 13904-1580 • USA
TELEPHONE: 1-800-HAWORTH (1-800-429-6784) / Outside US/Canada: (607) 722-5857
FAX: 1-800-895-0582 / Outside US/Canada: (607) 771-0012
E-mail to: orders@haworthpress.com

For orders outside US and Canada, you may wish to order through your local
sales representative, distributor, or bookseller.
For information, see http://haworthpress.com/distributors

(Discounts are available for individual orders in US and Canada only, not booksellers/distributors.)

PLEASE PHOTOCOPY THIS FORM FOR YOUR PERSONAL USE.
http://www.HaworthPress.com   BOF06